THE SPLENDOR OF TRUTH
AND
HEALTH CARE

Contributors to this Volume

E. Joanne Angelo, M.D.
Assistant Clinical Professor of Psychiatry
Tufts University School of Medicine
Boston, MA

Rev. Benedict Ashley, O.P.
Professor of Sacred Theology
Aquinas Institute of Theology
St. Louis, MO

Professor Gerard V. Bradley, B.A., J.D.
University of Notre Dame Law School
Notre Dame, IN

Nicholas P. Cafardi, Esq.
Dean of Law School
Duquesne University
Pittsburgh, PA

Patricia A. Cahill, J.D.
Executive Director
Alliance for Catholic Health
& Human Services
Archdiocese of New York

The Honorable Robert P. Casey
Governor
Commonwealth of Pennsylvania
Harrisburg, PA

Peter J. Cataldo, Ph.D.
Director of Research
Pope John Center
Braintree, MA

Rev. Romanus Cessario, O.P., S.T.L., S.T.D.
Professor of Sacred Theology
Dominican House of Studies
Washington, D.C.

Mr. Richard M. Doerflinger, M.A.Div.
Associate Director for Policy Development
Secretariat for Pro-Life Activities
National Conference of Catholic Bishops
Washington, DC

The Most Rev. Francis E. George, O.M.I.
Bishop of Yakima
Yakima, WA

Rev. Benedict J. Groeschel, C.F.R.
Office for Spiritual Development
Archdiocese of New York
Larchmont, NY

Professor Russell Hittinger, Ph. D.
806 Brompton Street
Fredericksburg, VA

Rev. Germain Kopaczynski, O.F.M. Conv.
Director of Education
Pope John Center
Braintree, MA

Ralph McInerny, Ph.D.
The Michael P. Grace Professor of
   Medieval Studies
Director of The Jacques Maritain Center
University of Notre Dame
Notre Dame, IN

Sr. Frances Marie Masching, O.S.F.
President
OSF Healthcare System
Peoria, IL

The Most Rev. John H. Ricard, S.S.J.
Auxiliary Bishop of Baltimore
Office of Urban Vicar
Baltimore, MD

Rev. Russell E. Smith, S.T.D.
President
Pope John Center
Braintree, MA

THE SPLENDOR OF TRUTH
AND
HEALTH CARE

Proceedings of the
Fourteenth Workshop for Bishops
Dallas, Texas

Russell E. Smith
Editor

*Publication of the Proceedings
was made possible
through a generous grant
from*
Mr. & Mrs. John A. McNeice, Jr.

The Pope John Center

Nihil Obstat: Rev. James A. O'Donohoe, J.C.D.

Imprimatur: Bernard Cardinal Law

Date: August 23, 1995

The Nihil Obstat and Imprimatur are a declaration that a book or pamphlet is considered to be free from doctrinal or moral error. It is not implied that those who have granted the Nihil Obstat and Imprimatur agree with the contents, opinions or statements expressed.

LIBRARY OF CONGRESS CATALOGING-IN-PUBLICATION DATA

Workshop for Bishops of the United States and Canada (14th : 1995 : Dallas, Tex.)
 The splendor of truth and health care : proceedings of the Fourteenth Bishops' Workshop, Dallas, Texas.
  p. cm. –(Catholic tradition and bioethics : 1)
  Includes bibliographical references.
  ISBN 0-935372-39-3 (paper)
 1. Medical ethics–Congresses. 2. Medicine–Religious aspects–Catholic Church–Congresses. 3. Catholic Church–Doctrines–Congresses. 4. Christian ethics–Catholic authors–Congresses. 5. Catholic Church. Pope (1978- : John Paul II). Veritatis splendor–Congresses. I. Title. II. Series.
R725.56.W67   1995   95-39696
174' .2–dc20   CIP

Contents

"Something Old, Something New"

This volume marks the end of one thing and the beginning of another. It is the end of the Workshop Proceedings as such and the beginning next year of an annual volume entitled *Studies in Catholic Tradition and Bioethics*. The annual volume will contain many of the talks of the Dallas Workshop for Bishops, but will also publish invited papers which are not part of the Workshops.

For some years, there has been a desire at the Pope John Center to produce something more substantial than the newsletter *Ethics & Medics* on a regular basis. A journal was suggested—monthly, bi-monthly or quarterly—as was an annual volume of essays that may either have one theme or varied topics in bioethics. On the other hand, it was felt that not to print at least some of the talks of the Dallas

Workshop for Bishops would constitute a squandering of precious resources.

After much discussion and many staff meetings, the idea of an annual volume was arrived at. While the Bishops' Workshop would generate the bulk of the articles, other articles would be invited which would not have been presented in Dallas and which in fact may not relate directly to the theme of the Workshop. This would allow most of the Dallas presentations to have a wider audience and it would provide the fruit of additional scholarship on topical subjects. Also, an article is foreseen that will present a round-up of the year in the field of bioethics from the perspective of Catholic moral theology. In the course of the next year, an Editorial Board will be assembled which will oversee the contents of these future volumes. In this way, the Pope John Center can make an even greater contribution to the tradition of Catholic bioethics.

The John A. and Margarete McNeice, Jr., Foundation

In addition to this, the Pope John Center is pleased to announce a new foundation that has been established to endow much of the research which will take place at the Center. Mr. John A. McNeice, Jr., of Boston has generously created the John A. and Margarete McNeice, Jr., Foundation. This foundation is directed at task force studies, publications, and consultation services, particularly those involving the salvific meaning of human suffering and vexing questions of conscience. The goal of the research which this foundation endows is ultimately to enable people to seek and to understand the Church's teaching of morality as a mission of God's mercy and a means to peace of mind. All of us at the Center are most grateful for the generosity of the McNeice family.

The Present Volume

This present volume contains the Proceedings of the fourteenth Workshop for Bishops in Dallas, Texas. The theme of the 1995 Workshop was "The Splendor of Truth and Health Care." Three documents of the teaching Church served as a framework for the deliberations animating the 1995 Bishops' Workshop. The first was the encyclical of the Supreme Pastor, Pope John Paul II's *The Splendor of Truth*; the second was a document of the Church Universal, *The Catechism of the Catholic Church*; the third was the ongoing effort of the Catholic Bishops of the United States of America to explain in an American setting the concerns of the Church for a morally adequate health care delivery system in the *Ethical and Religious Directives for Catholic Health Care Services*. The aim of the Workshop was two-fold: first, to foster a deeper understanding of these three valuable doctrinal resources, and second, to impart pastoral insights regarding how these documents may be used as tools for evangelization.

Bishop Francis E. George, O.M.I., delivered the Keynote address entitled "Bishops and the Splendor of Public Truth." A major theme in the encyclical *Veritatis Splendor* is that law and freedom are not opposed to each other. Their harmony was addressed by Professor Russell Hittinger. A second major theme, addressed by Father Romanus Cessario, O.P., is the question of moral absolutes as a guarantor of an authentically human and truly just community. The role of exceptionless moral norms in safeguarding human happiness was examined, focusing upon unchanging moral values as one of the building blocks of a sound anthropology, one based on Christian values, to be sure, yet also serviceable for the entire human community.

There follow three presentations on practical issues in health care ethics: uterine isolation/tubal ligation (Father Germain Kopaczynski, O.F.M. Conv.), recent legislation regarding health care reform initiatives (Richard Doerflinger), and canonical issues for Catholic health care sponsors (Dean Nicholas Cafardi).

Two major talks were devoted to the *Catechism of the Catholic Church*. How are bishops to teach the truth of Christ in an age that lives for the moment? How is the Gospel to reach and change the hearts of people raised in such an age? Father Benedict Ashley, O.P., addresses himself to the development of moral doctrine, that ability of the Church to be a pilgrim through the centuries, to live in history, and yet continue to teach the timeless saving message of Jesus Christ, "the same yesterday, today, and forever." This is followed by Professor Ralph McInerny's examination of our age and the Church's response to it found in the *Catechism*. While our age may be bewitched by Pilate's question, "What is truth?" the Church in her teaching affirms that moral relativism is not the final word. She does so by continuing to bear witness to the truth of Christ's words: "I am the Way, the Truth and the Life." In the best Catholic tradition, while the *Catechism* is certainly a work of its era, its main message is to challenge the mores of the age. The task of evangelization demands nothing less.

Next follow three presentations of timely concern: women and health care (Joanne Angelo, M.D.), evangelizing for morality (Father Benedict Groeschel, C.F.R.) and an overview of the 1994 revision of the *Ethical and Religious Directives.*

Professor of Law Gerald Bradley treated the constitutional question occasioned by the new health care climate, namely, whether Catholic health care professionals and facilities can continue to provide quality health care according to the teachings of the Church. This issue is not one of interest only to Catholics; in more ways than one, the very health of the nation is at stake, involving as it does the conscience of the nation. It is not only bishops who must face the challenge of evangelizing in the modern world; it is a challenge facing faith-filled politicians as well. Former Governor of Pennsylvania Robert P. Casey's essay deals with the role that faith plays in animating one's political convictions, attempting to illustrate how to bring the values of a living faith into an often unbelieving public arena.

Finally, the issues of what should be included and excluded in a basic health care benefits package is addressed by Bishop John Richard, S.S.J. Perhaps in no other area of concern over competing health care proposals which took place all over America from 1992 to 1994 was there a need for the richness of Catholic moral reflection to be brought to bear than on the proper response to this question. Also of concern for Catholic sponsors and providers of health care is the moral evaluation of health care alliances which was addressed by me with responses by Sister Frances Marie Masching, O.S.F., President of the

O.S.F. Health Care System in Peoria, and Patricia A. Cahill, J.D., Director of Health and Hospitals for the Archdiocese of New York.

* * *

As is true for each of the Bishops' Workshops, many people contributed generously to the successful execution of the 1995 Workshop for Bishops. The planning, content, and hospitality necessary for an international event of this magnitude depend on many hard-working, self-sacrificing individuals who obviously love the Church very much. We are very grateful to everyone who made this Workshop such a success.

We are especially grateful to the Supreme Knight, Mr. Virgil C. Dechant, and to the Knights of Columbus for their generous sponsorship of this workshop. We are grateful as well to the faculty of presenters assembled for this gathering, for their patience with the many deadlines and for their scholarly competence and presentations.

Special thanks go to the Most Reverend Charles V. Grahmann, Bishop of Dallas, for his gracious hospitality. Thanks also to the seminarians of the Diocese of Dallas who are home on their "pastoral year" for serving the Masses, singing, and acting as sacristans. In this regard, special thanks go to Father Thomas Cloherty for overseeing all the liturgical arrangements. We are also very grateful to the local councils of the Knights of Columbus and the Catholic Women's Guilds of the Diocese of Dallas for their kind assistance. Thanks also to the Spanish translators—Fathers Rutilio J. del Riego and Rolando Fonseca and Sister Margarita Cecilia Velez, O.P., from Texas, and Sister M. Nieves, P.D.D.M., from the Archdiocese of Boston.

We are also grateful to the staff of the Harvey Hotel in Addison for their graciousness and service. A very special word of thanks goes to the Nuns of the Poor Clare Federation of Mary Immaculate, the Daughters of St. Paul, and the Sisters of Charity of Convent Station in the city of Boston and their grammar school children who prayed for the success and for the participants of the conference.

As mentioned above, we are most grateful to Mr. John A. McNeice, Jr., whose foundation provides the funding for this publication.

Finally, we are deeply grateful to Mrs. Jeanne Burke and Mr. Donald Powers for their indefatigable effort and diligent assistance from the beginning of this workshop's conception to the moment this book was delivered to your hands.

The Reverend Russell E. Smith, S.T.D.
President
Feast of the Most Sacred Heart of Jesus
Boston, Massachusetts

To My Brother Bishops
Taking Part in the Fourteenth Workshop Organized
by the Pope John XXIII Medical-Moral Research
and Education Center

I greet you in the name of the Lord Jesus Christ as you come together for a week of study, reflection, and prayer. As Shepherds and Teachers of the Christian faithful in Canada, the Caribbean, Central America, Mexico, the Philippines, and the United States, you "come aside and rest a little" (cf. Mk 6:31) in the presence of the Lord who will enable you, in turn, to nourish the flock entrusted to you, with his word and the Sacraments. Once more the generosity of the Knights of Columbus has made it possible for the Pope John XXIII Medical-Moral Research and Education Center to organize this Workshop, the fourteenth in the series on medical-moral questions.

The theme of your Workshop, "The Splendor of Truth and Health Care," embraces a variety of topics and issues which involve your pastoral activity and teaching. In particular, modern health care presents delicate ethical and moral questions which require close attention and competent study on the part of the Church's Pastors. These questions are connected above all to the moral teaching of the Magisterium about the origin and transmission of human life, its inalienable dignity which must be respected and defended from the moment of conception to the moment of natural death, human sexuality and the techniques of the regulation of fertility. Two recent documents of the Magisterium will guide your reflection: the *Catechism of the Catholic Church*, which is a sure and authentic reference text for teaching

13

Catholic doctrine, and the Encyclical *Veritatis Splendor*, which deals with certain fundamental questions regarding the Church's moral teaching against the background of a questioning of traditional moral doctrine (cf. *Veritatis Splendor*, no. 4). I am confident that prayerful reflection on the contents of *Veritatis Splendor* will help you and your brother Bishops not only in applying the Church's moral doctrine to the new and emerging questions raised by advances in the various fields of medical science and technologies, but also in clarifying the anthropological and theological bases on which the Church's teaching stands.

The teachings of the Magisterium are normative for Catholic health facilities and are constitutive of their identity. It is this truth which engages the mission and pastoral responsibility of the Church's Pastors in a very personal way. A Bishop will always have to delegate certain responsibilities with regard to the *Catholic institutions* operating within his Diocese. But this does not relieve him of the personal obligation to watch over the faith and Christian life of his people and, where necessary, to call for proper teaching of the moral law (cf. VS, no. 116). I encourage you to use the opportunity afforded by the present Workshop to renew and reconfirm your commitment to this sacred duty.

May the Holy Spirit enlighten your minds and hearts as you consider and discuss topics of professional health-care practices, health-care reform, and therapeutic techniques. I entrust your reflections to the intercession of Mary, Mother of the Redeemer. May she bring you the riches of her Divine Son's graces. To all taking part in your Workshop I gladly impart my Apostolic Blessing.

From the Vatican, January 26, 1995

Joannes Paulus PP. II

Greetings from the Knights of Columbus

Virgil C. Dechant,
Supreme Knight

Your Eminences and Your Excellencies:

It is a pleasure and an honor to extend greetings on behalf of the Knights of Columbus to this Fourteenth Bishops' Workshop organized by the Pope John Center. With good reason, we consider this annual program to be among the most valuable and worthy of the many projects we support.

As you are well aware, loyal Catholic lay people look to you, their pastoral leaders, for informed, courageous guidance, faithful to the Church's authentic doctrine, on the many complex moral issues of the day. It is the hope and the belief of the Knights of Columbus that these workshops provide important help to you in meeting this responsibility.

The theme of this year's Workshop, "The Splendor of Truth and Health Care," promises sessions of great timeliness and relevance. Shaping a health care system that meets human needs and conforms to moral norms is an urgent challenge for the Church and society at large. In Pope John Paul's great encyclical, we have a cogent and comprehensive source of magisterial teaching to assist this effort.

In recent days, Bishop Daily and I had the great privilege of being with the Holy Father on the occasion of the World Youth Day in the Philippines. Once again we were reminded of—and deeply edified by—his uncompromising commitment to the dignity and sanctity of human life, as well as to the integrity of the received teaching of the Church.

No one hearing Pope John Paul, I believe, could help but recall his extraordinary defense of these values in the context of last year's international conference on population and development in Cairo. The intense hostility now directed against him in some quarters is a measure of his success.

This struggle, perhaps the most crucial of our times, goes on. It continues every day all around the world, and it may flare up with special intensity at the UN conference on women next September in Beijing. Ultimately, the issues at stake are the nature of the human person and the meaning of human life. Thank God we have the splendor of truth on our side! May it illuminate your deliberations in Dallas this week.

January 31, 1995
Dallas, Texas

Chapter 1

BISHOPS AND THE
SPLENDOR OF PUBLIC TRUTH

The Most Reverend Francis E. George, O.M.I.

1. Bishops as Teachers in *Veritatis Splendor*

Breaking what had become a pattern in recent encyclicals and papal messages, *Veritatis Splendor* is addressed not to the bishops, the faithful and all of good will but to the bishops and, only through them, to the whole Church and the general society. As teachers of the faith and therefore also of the way that leads to salvation, bishops confirm, support and counsel those who seek to better understand "moral demands in the areas of human sexuality, the family, and social economic and political life" (VS no. 4). *Veritatis Splendor*, however, is less directed to any of these particular questions, which every bishop addresses as occasion demands, than to the foundations of moral theology. This Encyclical is therefore both an aid and a challenge to our teaching ministry with and under Peter.

Bishops, both individually and collectively, have grown accustomed to speaking to the sins of individuals and of society: violence, abortion, polymorphous sexual activity, unjust profits and wages, the morality of war or of a nuclear deterrent, the various moral questions that arise in health care and its delivery; but we do not often speak to the bases of moral theory, to the intellectual foundations of the praxis which is shaped by and protects the faith. To do so brings us into dialogue with ethicists and moral theologians, as the Pope engages them in Chapter Two of *Veritatis Splendor*, and with the shapers of our culture, as the Pope engages them in Chapter Three of the Encyclical. These are daunting conversations, and we might be excused for listening and meditating without joining the conversation ourselves. Episcopal irenicism arises often from a genuinely pastoral concern to be what a bishop must be: a center of unity, a man of contacts, around whom all can gather who want to gather in Christ, a man of dialogue who rejects no one and is respectful of all opinions.

The Pope himself is such a bishop, but he is more and he challenges us to be more. At a moment in history when the human race seems to be at a turning point, the Holy Father asks us to speak the truth precisely as bishops: "We have the duty, as Bishops, to be vigilant that the word of God is faithfully taught. My Brothers in the Episcopate, it is part of our pastoral ministry to see to it that this moral teaching is faithfully handed down and to have recourse to appropriate measures to ensure that the faithful are guarded from every doctrine and theory contrary to it. In carrying out this task we are all assisted by theologians; even so, theological opinions constitute neither the rule nor the norm of our teaching. Its authority is derived, by the assistance of the Holy Spirit and in communion *cum Petro et sub Petro*, from our fidelity to the Catholic faith which comes from the Apostles. As Bishops, we have the grave obligation to be *personally* vigilant that the 'sound doctrine' (1 Tim. 1:10) of faith and morals is taught in our Dioceses" (VS no. 116).

2. The Loss of Public Truth:
The Problem of Shaping Moral Conversations

Can we speak the truth today? People say all kinds of things and proclaim all kinds of opinions. Some of it is bound to be true! What is difficult to say publicly is that what we say about morality is, in fact, the truth. The claim to speak the truth about moral questions is resented and makes whatever particular judgments we make more difficult to hear.

One of the reasons *Veritatis Splendor* expends so much effort in connecting truth and freedom is because objective moral truth is now often regarded as a threat to subjective personal freedom. In the United States, the Church can speak to the Gospel meaning of freedom. Freedom is our major cultural value, and even the Church can talk about what it should mean. We can, as well, reexamine the demands of evangelical justice, because justice is another cultural value. Even when U.S. citizens recognize the deficiencies of our theories of justice and our failure to act justly, justice remains a public imperative. The Church can figure in conversations around it and help change institutions and structures. But there are few resources in our culture to express and explain the demands of the Gospel as true, because religious truth is no longer a public virtue. "Any truth not immediately verifiable in observation or through the methodologies of the hard sciences becomes private opinion. It enters the public realm under the rubric of personal expression, a value which is the subject of arbitration but not of intellectual research."[1] The public authority, the government, while it must protect freedom and foster justice, is not supposed to teach any particular truth. But the Church must; and this claim to teach the truth is truly counter-cultural. How, then, can we teach the truth about the way that leads to human happiness? What language is available? What allies can we find?

The Pope's discussion of the relation between truth and freedom is rooted in his anthropology.[2] As a phenomenologist, he brings from experience the distinction between "I act" and "Something is happening in me." This distinction enables us to recognize within ourselves the difference between person and nature. The transcendence of the person shows itself in the liberty of willed action; but we integrate our emotional life, what happens to us, into our freedom as each of us judges and chooses which values to act upon, which to implement in our lives. Moral conscience, if it is not reduced to pure willfulness, is the place where personal transcendence shows itself in act. But the person's transcendence of nature cannot betray or run counter to the person's own specific and shared nature. Each person must act, and thereby create his or her personal identity; but each must act according to the truth of things, lest the personal identity created in acting be monstrous. As Newman saw, conscience is less a *rule* of right conduct than it is a *sanction* of right conduct.[3] When we act against our nature, personal conscience stings. Conscience guides each person to his or her full development; but this development is fulfilled by placing oneself at the service of others. Why? Because the nature of the human person is fulfilled in the generosity which makes him or her the image of an infinitely generous, self-sacrificing God.

Obviously, with that last sentence, the papal anthropology moves from philosophical anthropology to a notion that comes to us from historical revelation. This integration of the truths of natural reason, to use the classical phrase, and the truths of revelation in John Paul's anthropology shows up in the Encyclical when he mixes in one list acts classified as intrinsically evil from either source (VS nos. 80 and 81) and when he begins the Encyclical with a meditation upon a passage from the Gospel according to St. Matthew. To find objective truth, human or moral truth, for the sake of genuine personal freedom, we are directed first to look at Christ rather than at nature. Coming to know and love Christ, we find the love necessary to give up our personal freedom for the sake of the truth that sets us free to sacrifice ourselves for others. In that act of generosity, we both establish personally and discover naturally the truth which leads us back to Christ as his disciples, even unto death.

The Pope's integration of metaphysics and phenomenology in his anthropology, the blending of philosophy and theology in his moral teaching, the intertwining of critical reason and faith in his use of Sacred Scripture tend to infuriate the specialists in each domain. Nevertheless, it has given him a language to preach and to persuade, a public language which reaches over the heads of those who claim to own a discipline to the people of faith and others of good will who want to hear the truth, even if they don't always like what they hear.

The Pope, himself a creative scholar, respects and cherishes scholarship in any field. The sophistication of his own mind, however, leads him to recognize that the very methodologies which advance a science and are necessary to its progress also limit it.

It seems to me we have here a case of war being too important to be left to generals, the Bible being too basic to be left to scripture scholars, morals being too central to be left to professional ethicists. Any argument must be appropriately criticized, including those put forth by the Pope; but genuine intellectual sophistication does not stop with a single scholarly critique of the faith. It continues with a critique of the critique, not to re-establish an unjustified or naive faith but to enter into what contemporary hermeneuticist Paul Ricoeur has called "second naivete." Just as important, however, as the papal argument, which will be presented to us and criticized in the course of the next few days, is the papal example. John Paul II is finding "ever new ways of speaking with love and mercy" (VS no. 3), and so must we.

3. Finding a Language for Public Discussion of Moral Issues: Objective Truth in Natural Law

Paradoxically, the Encyclical's emphasis on natural law as central to the Church's moral teaching often seems more a hindrance than a help in finding a public language for conversation on moral questions today.

A. CLASSICAL DEDUCTIVE NATURAL LAW THEORY

As we all know, the Church has borrowed elements of classical natural law theory and incorporated them into her teaching. Thomas Aquinas in his treatise on law in the *Summa Theologiae* (I-II, Q.90) listed natural moral law as one of four kinds of law, the three others being God's eternal law and human and divine positive law. Eternal law is God's plan for the world, the purpose encoded in creation itself by the Creator. The Divine Reason or purpose can therefore be known by human creatures through reasoning about the goals or ends of things, their intrinsic purposes. Early scientific methodology was more observation than experimentation, like attending a basketball game and writing the rule book by watching how the players move and interact in order to achieve the goal of the game. In some cosmologies, both ancient and modern, purpose is as much in every part of nature as intention is in every woman or man. We read the laws of nature by observing how things act and thereby discovering why they act. The human person's ability to intend something freely, even to put nature at cross-purposes to itself, establishes human nature's specificity and enables rational creatures to participate in divine providence. To understand our nature, we read our basic inclinations and deduce from them the principles or premises of natural law for human moral activity.

This short recall is enough for remembering also the difficulties in using natural law theory in public discussions today. The meaning of nature has changed. It is not an intrinsic, purposive principle of operation, encompassing even human nature and the divine nature; it is instead a purely physical matrix for manipulation by humans who define themselves against nature rather than as part of it. The new ecological consciousness, in approaching nature as a museum piece to be preserved rather than a field to be exploited, does not really reduce the modern distance between nature and man.

The meaning of law has changed too. It is less "an ordinance of reason for the common good" (Aquinas) than a statistical generality in nature or a jointly willed consensus in human community. Since the meaning of law has changed, natural law theory seems vacuous and *a priori*. It is not shaped by human desires, any more than physical nature itself is so shaped, and it is hard to understand how its premises can be useful in judging, for example, positive laws passed by a legislature.

Natural law continues to bury its undertakers, however, because the positive laws we live under raise questions which positive law cannnot answer: is this law just or unjust? Should an unjust law be obeyed? What tells us that a legal system as such is good or bad? Are there limits that can never be crossed, actions that can never be justified, no matter what positive law says or doesn't say? How can we judge the law itself?

B. Dialogical Natural Law Theory in *Veritatis Splendor*

Perhaps in an effort to ground natural law theory in a less deductive and more experiential methodology, John Paul II uses the Gospel dialogue between Jesus and the rich young man about what it means to do good to illustrate how the dynamics of self-discovery become the dynamics of conversion to Christ. The task of obeying the commandments, both those of Sinai and those of nature, becomes the joy of discovering, in Christ, the moral good which satisfies all our natural longings.

Behind this dialogical approach to a discovery of what human nature tells us about human morality are Karol Wojtyla's analyses of intersubjectivity. Genuinely human intersubjectivity comes into our experience only if we can move progressively through bonds of sentiment, false idealism and even true comradeship to a mutual personal surrender, in which what is deepest in both persons, their subjectivity, becomes united in a love which takes them both beyond themselves. Karol Wojtyla analyzed meticulously the stages of knowing and loving in discussing human sexuality,[4] which becomes a language proclaiming God's purposes. The same model of analysis, however, enters into other moral arguments. To the traditional study of the sources of morality in the right ordering of the object of the act, its circumstances and the moral agent's intention, John Paul II adds an analysis of the acting subject naturally ordered to the goodness of God made visible in Christ and therefore called, from within, to act freely in co-natural conformity to the very highest good. To discover natural moral law, the human moral agent enters into dialogue with his or her own nature as uncovered in responsible action. The end of such action is, however, the happiness that can be ours only in the embrace of God's goodness. Acts intrinsically disordered, i.e., acts unable to be ordered to God, unable to be performed in God's presence, destroy both the objective moral order and the subject performing them.[5]

They also destroy moral community. Our common attraction to goods which are ordered to God and which are achieved or lost through our actions is the foundation not only of personal happiness but also of human solidarity and ecclesial communion. The sense that this is so leads many even outside the household of the faith to be open to John Paul's project without fully accepting his argument. Many, for example, would applaud the Pope's insistence that there are absolute moral principles, without accepting his argument on intrinsically evil acts. This is an opening that should be welcomed. Despite the difficulties inherent in the use of natural law for public discussion, might we bishop-conversationalists find in it a bridge, perhaps a narrow bridge, to other moral traditions in today's society? Two groups with whom it would be useful to ally, if possible, in the public discussion of moral issues are secularists and evangelicals.

C. Shards of Natural Law Theory in Empiricist Culture: A Bridge to Secularists?

A generation ago, Fr. John Courtney Murray tried very hard to rework the natural law vocabulary of the United States' founding documents in order to use it once again as a language of public discourse for this country. If natural law language were comprehensible to society at large, it would delineate the Church's common ground with secularists in moral conversation. The John Courtney Murray project, as it is now called, continues because it offers hope for a common moral language.[6]

Natural law at the time of the United States' political formation was natural law as interpreted by Thomas Hobbes and John Locke. Unfortunately, the natural state of man for both philosophers was bereft of government and other social institutions. These were founded on a social contract rather than on the political nature of man. But the social contract only saves people from the worst in themselves; and justice, in social contract theories, is less a positive good than a necessary evil. It protects natural rights to life, liberty and property but does not give positive guidelines for achieving a just society. Nor does natural law theory in English empiricism establish laws for personal conduct. For these, Locke fell back on utilitarian theory.

Whether because of Locke or because of the entrepreneurial attitudes necessary for creating a continent-wide nation in less than a century, the United States is largely a nation of utilitarians or even of moral pragmatists. We argue more readily from consequences than from principles. Modern pragmatic philosophers have, nevertheless, tried various ways to derive from experience itself, even the experience of nature, general ethical imperatives and moral laws.

Empiricists concerned with moral theory ask: how is it possible to derive an "ought" from an "is"? How do we find in present experience the norms to judge this and future experience morally? Most American empiricists who have tried to create an empiricist natural law theory have depended on some form of emergent probability as an explanation of the natural cosmos. From the continuum of temporal experience, some moments are qualitatively as well as quantitatively different from others, such that they begin to function as norms for other experiences. Usually these more valuable experiences are full of personal satisfaction, or they are able to unite other experiences and give them meaning, or they make possible a qualitative leap in evolution. The passage from fact to norm is piloted by value, but this sort of moral theory usually founders on the definition of value. Current public discussion about values makes the difficulty clear.[7]

Anglican missionary and theologian Lesslie Newbigin makes of the modern distinction between values and facts the primary obstacle for preaching the Gospel in modern societies. When facts are public and values are private, the chasm between them cannot be closed and the Gospel is so relativized that it loses its effectiveness.[8] Bringing the fact/value distinction itself into public discussion today would help turn the current concern about returning values to public schools and public life into a more basic conversation about how our culture shortchanges human intellectuality itself, depriving it of its natural openness to transcendent reality and reducing it to a mere means for plotting individual objectives. Nonetheless, such a discussion seems unlikely. Some intellectual conversions presuppose the very moral and religious conversions they are supposed to foster. In order for faith to seek understanding from philosophical moral theories, theorists have to believe in order to understand. The clash is one of wills before it is a war of intellects.

25

D. NATURAL LAW THEORY AND BIBLICAL LANGUAGE: A BRIDGE TO EVANGELICALS?

The language of religious conversion is natural to evangelicals, and perhaps that partially explains current efforts to ally ourselves with them on issues of public morality in this country.[9] Theoretically, however, while evangelicals are open to legal theories which presuppose a creator God, as does classical natural law theory, and are willing to explore moral responsibility apart from explicit belief in Jesus Christ, as affirmed by St. Paul in the first chapter of Romans, the noetic consequences of Adam's fall render natural law theory impossible to formulate and idolatrous to the extent it subordinates divine revelation to human reason in discovering universal ethical standards.[10] Not nature but God's Kingdom is morally normative. John Paul II, who helped author *Gaudium et Spes*, obviously enjoys using the language of each to enhance our understanding of both. Evangelicals who will welcome chapter one of *Veritatis Splendor*, however, will receive chapter two with only slightly less caution than some of our own moral theologians. Nevertheless, the encyclical is itself a welcome occasion for bishops to dialogue with all.

4. Moral Issues and the New Evangelization

Focusing however quickly on the need for intellectual, moral and religious conversion in order to converse about public morality brings us to the same end as *Veritatis Splendor* itself: the moral life in the context of the new evangelization. The specificity of the new evangelization, I would argue, is less the recognition that mission is now on all continents or that there are sociological groupings and whole professions still unaffected by the Gospel, than it is the recognition in sorrow that there are entire cultures once Christian which now stand in need of conversion to Christ. For many once Christian peoples today, the Gospel is neither good nor news.

While it is harder to preach to those who have effectively rejected the Gospel than to those who have never heard it, the deficiencies and neediness of many cultures provide an opening for evangelizers. Contemporary neediness is two-fold, according to the Pope: the need for God's love and the need for secure moral standards. The goals of the new evangelization, therefore, are to share, with respect for all peoples, a sense of God's transcendence and a secure ethical base (VS no. 107). Neither of these can be shared except by people who live in hope and who can give reason for the hope that is in them (1 Peter 3, 15-6).

In a pragmatic, future-oriented culture, secularists believe in measurable progress and evangelicals calculate Christ's imminent return. But the Enlightenment paradigm for understanding human nature, even though it has its fortresses in newsrooms and classrooms and still shapes our public life, is philosophically exhausted. The Fundamentalist, if not the evangelical, understanding of life in Christ is less than adequate in introducing people to the whole Christ and fails to respect the work of the Spirit outside of a narrow evangelism. Perhaps dialogue with both can begin with the love that grounds our hope, even if our words are less than adequate. There is a logic of love which continues to speak of hope, even when words fail.

If we continue to search for words to preach a Christ who is clearly the transcendent God become one of us for our salvation and if we witness from within our own cultures to the way that leads to a share in Christ's own goodness, the Churches shepherded by us will be beacons of hope, not just for individuals but for entire societies. The splendor of moral truth is not fully public today, but neither is it hidden under a bushel basket. In encouraging one another through meetings such as this, we will find ways to implement the Pope's program, which is Christ's, even if at times we need arguments and a language somewhat different from his.

Notes

1. Francis E. George, "Evangelizing American Culture," in Kenneth Boyack, *The New Catholic Evangelization* (New York: Paulist, 1991), 53.

2. See Antoine Guggenheim, "Liberté et vérité selon K. Wojtyla," *Nouvelle Revue Theologique*, 115 (1993): 400-411; Karol Wojtyla, *The Acting Person*, translated by Andrzej Potocki (Dordrecht, Holland: D. Reidel, 1979), chapter 3.

3. See John Henry Newman, *An Essay in Aid of a Grammar of Assent* (London: Longmans, Green and Co., 1903), 106.

4. See Karol Wojtyla, *Love and Responsibility*, translated by H.T. Willetts (New York: Farrar, Straus, Giroux, 1981). For a more general analysis of intersubjectivity

in action, see Karol Wojtyla, *The Acting Person*, chapters five and six, and Karol Wojtyla, "The Person: Subject and Community," *Review of Metaphysics* 33 (1979): 273-308.

5. See Francis E. George, "Teaching Moral Theology in the Light of the Dialogical Framework of *Veritatis Splendor*," *Seminarium* XXXIV (1994): n. 1, 43-51.

6. See Paul J. Weithman, "John Courtney Murray—Do His Ideas Still Matter?" *America* (Oct. 29, 1994): 17-21; the English language edition of the international theology review *Communio* has carried numerous articles by David Schindler, Michael Novak and Joseph Komonchak addressing both the value and the proper interpretation of Fr. Murray's work.

7. John Dewey and Josiah Royce, using very different metaphysical systems, both sought to discover moral norms, even for individuals, in social experience. This strain of American pragmatic theory might be explored more thoroughly by bishops trying to find bases for dialogue on natural law in American culture. Through his writing on the Beloved Community, Royce has also influenced American social theory and social activists such as Martin Luther King, Jr. For Royce's influence on interpretation theory, see Robert S. Corrington, *The Community of Interpreters: on the Hermeneutics of Nature and the Bible in the American Philosophical Tradition* (Macon, GA: Mercer University Press, 1987).

8. Lesslie Newbigin, *Foolishness to the Greeks: the Gospel and Western Culture* (Grand Rapids: Eerdmans, 1986).

9. See William Bentley Ball, ed., *In Search of a National Morality: a Manifesto for Evangelicals and Catholics* (Grand Rapids, Baker Book House, 1992) and "Evangelicals and Catholics Together: A Declaration," *First Things* (May, 1994): 15-22.

10. See Carl F. H. Henry, "Natural Law and a Nihilistic Culture," *First Things* (Jan., 1995): 54-60.

Chapter 2

LAW AND LIBERTY IN
VERITATIS SPLENDOR

Russell Hittinger, Ph.D.

I

One of the most curious and disturbing trends of our culture is the belief that the chief purpose of law is to annul the law itself. When authority is used to divest the community of its obligations under law, or when authority is used to recognize rights as so many immunities against the law—indeed when authority is used to subvert authority—then we tend to say that law is good, which is to say that it is accomplishing humane ends. Our ecclesial culture does not remain unaffected by this attitude. Issues of moral theology are invariably reduced to questions of authority. When the Pope said that he has no authority to ordain women, many Catholics and non-Catholics alike were shocked by the suggestion that the Pope cannot use law for any purpose he so pleases. Whether we are speaking of marriage tribunals, altar girls, holy days of obligation, contraception, public policy on abortion, or whatever, people inside and outside the Church want you to use your apostolic authority to ratify the liberty of individual choice. Law, it seems, is but a malleable tool in the hands of an interpreting community. When it binds, it is called legalism; when it loosens, it is praised as humane.[1]

The Pope speaks to this problem at the very outset of *Veritatis Splendor*, when he recounts the colloquy between Jesus and the rich young man in Mt. 19.

> Then someone came to him and said, "Teacher, what good must I do to have eternal life?" And he said to him, "Why do you ask me about what is good? There is only one who is good. If you wish to enter into life, keep the commandments." He said to him, "Which ones?" And Jesus said, "You shall not murder; You shall not commit adultery; You shall not steal; You shall not bear false witness; Honour your father and mother; also, You shall love your neighbor as yourself." The young man said to him, "I have kept all these; what do I still lack?" Jesus said to him, "If you wish to be perfect, go, sell your possessions and give the money to the poor, and you will have treasure in heaven; then come, follow me." (VS no. 6)

The Pope explains that the first and ultimate question of morality is not a lawyerly question. Unlike the Pharisees, the rich young man does not ask what the bottom line is, from a legal standpoint. Rather, he asks what must be done in order to achieve the unconditional good, which is communion with God. Christ takes the sting out of law, not by annulling it, but by revealing the Good to which it directs us. Remove or forget the Good and it is inevitable that law becomes legalism. Legalism is nothing other than law without its context.

30

The scripture relates that the young man went away sad, for he had many possessions. But the modern audience is more apt to turn away sad when faced with the teaching that there is a moral law that is indispensable, and indeed which binds authority itself. The Pope sometimes is treated like a simpleton, an ecclesiastical version of Dan Quayle, when he points out that all issues of circumstance, culture, place and time notwithstanding, certain actions can never be made right, and that no human "law" can make them right. Just as from the scales and axiomatic measures of music there can come a Beethoven sonata, or a Penderecki 12-tone composition, so too from obedience to the commandments there opens the possibility of a creative, fluid, and completely realized human liberty. The point of learning the scales is not mindless repetition; the point is to make beautiful music. No doubt, a piano teacher who only focused upon the scales would be a simpleton, a legalist as it were. But a piano teacher who neglected to call the pupil's attention to the scalar rudiments would not be worthy of the name teacher. Musical order does not, and indeed cannot, begin merely with human spontaneity and creative improvisation. The same is true in the domain of moral action. Any one who would set up an opposition between law and freedom, and then take the side of freedom, not only under-estimates the need for law, but misrepresents the nature of freedom.

The story of the rich young man, of course, shows the essential unity of the Law and Gospel. In *Veritatis* the Pope also spends considerable effort in dealing with a related theme: namely, the unity of the two tables of the Decalogue. "Acknowledging the Lord as God," he says, "is the very core, the heart of the law, from which the particular precepts flow and toward which they are ordered" (VS no. 11). Each precept, he continues, "is the interpretation of what the words 'I am the Lord your God' mean for man" (VS no. 13).

This morning I shall focus upon the issue of the two tables because it not only situates the theme of law and freedom, but it also stands at the center of the dispute between the Pope and the dissenting moral theologians. The terms of this dispute require very technical philosophical discussion, which cannot be rehearsed here at its proper level of detail and complexity. But we can spend a few minutes considering the theological ground of the problem. The ground of the problem is actually quite simple, so simple in fact that it is easy to overlook it, or to mistake it for some other kind of problem.

II

Question: Upon creation, did God give to our first parents a kind of plenary authority over "ethics"—over a sphere of this worldly conduct that more or less corresponds to the second table of the Decalogue? In *Veritatis*, the Pope has this to say about the answer often given by moral theologians:

> Some people...disregarding the dependence of human reason on Divine Wisdom...have actually posited a "complete sovereignty of reason" in the domain of moral norms regarding the right ordering of life in this world. Such norms would constitute the boundaries for a merely "human" morality; they would be the expression of a law which man in an autonomous manner lays down for himself and which has its source exclusively in human reason. In no way could God be considered the Author of this law, except in the sense that human reason exercises its autonomy in setting down laws by virtue of a primordial and total mandate given to man by God. These trends of thought have led to a denial, in opposition to Sacred Scripture (cf. Mt 15:3-6) and the Church's constant teaching, of the fact that the natural moral law has God as its author, and that man, by the use of reason, participates in the eternal law, which it is not for him to establish. (VS no. 36)

"[C]ertain moral theologians," the Pope continues, "have introduced a sharp distinction, contrary to Catholic doctrine, between an 'ethical order,' which would be human in origin and of value for 'this world' alone, and an 'order of salvation' for which only certain intentions and interior attitudes regarding God and neighbor would be significant. This has then led to an actual denial that there exists, in Divine Revelation, a specific and determined moral content, universally valid and permanent. The word of God would be limited to proposing an exhortation...which the autonomous reason alone would then have the task of completing with normative directives which are truly 'objective,' that is, adapted to the concrete historical situation" (VS no. 37).

32

Notice that the Pope does not accuse these (unnamed) theologians of proposing that some moral norms are naturally known, even by people who are ignorant of revelation. The Catholic church has always held that some rudimentary precepts of the natural law are known naturally, without instruction afforded by divine positive law. Instead, the Pope accuses certain unnamed theologians of constructing a sphere of human moral choice independent of, and immune from, divine governance. The fact that the human mind is naturally competent to make moral judgments is construed to mean that the human practical reason has dominion. From the premise that the human mind has a natural, jurisdictional dominion over "ethics," it would seem to follow that the Church ought to butt out, and use its offices only as a kind of bully pulpit for exhorting the otherwise autonomous human agent. However, for the Church to butt out of "ethics," it will be necessary to get God out of the picture. Some theologians remove God from the picture by arguing that, at creation, God removed Himself. It was God, after all, who created human practical reason, endowing it with a natural competence over moral conduct. By emphasizing human jurisdictional authority over ethics, these theologians perhaps do not go so far as Marcion, for they do not posit an absolute dualism between creation and salvation, or between law and Gospel. Their opinion more resembles the modern Deistic theology, according to which God indeed creates, and what He creates is good; but He hands over jurisdiction of creation to the human mind.

Thus we find Father Joseph Fuchs contending in his most recent book that: "When in fact, nature-creation does speak to us, it tells us only what it is and how it functions on its own. In other words, the Creator shows us what is divinely willed to exist, and how it functions, but not how the Creator wills the human being qua person to use this existing reality."[2] Fuchs goes on to assert that: "Neither the Hebrew Bible nor the new Testament produces statements that are independent of culture and thus universal and valid for all time; nor can these statements be given by the church or its magisterium. Rather, it is the task of human beings—of the various persons who have been given the requisite intellectual capacity—to investigate what can and must count as a conviction about these responsibilities."[3] In other words, God creates, but he gives no operating instructions. The natural norm will have to be drawn from human reason; or, as Fuchs suggests, those "who have been given the requisite intellectual capacity." I take this to mean academic ethicians and moral theologians.

We should not overlook the fact that this kind of theology was prominent in the dissent of the theologians against *Humanæ Vitæ*. The majority of Paul VI's Commission for the Study of Problems of the Family, Population, and Birth Rate issued a report urging that the Church change her teaching on contraception. The authors of the majority report at least had the honesty to clearly state their theological premise. They reasoned that although the sources of human life are from created nature, the rules for the choice and administration of that natural value fall to human jurisdiction. "To take his own or another's life is a sin," the Majority Report contended, "not because life is under the exclusive dominion of God but because it is contrary to right reason unless there is question of a good or a higher order."[4]

Similarly, Father Fuchs asserts that: "One cannot…deduce, from God's relationship to creation, what the obligation of the human person is in these areas or in the realm of creation as a whole."[5] Regarding *Gaudium et Spes*, where the human conscience is spoken of as a *sacrarium* in which we find ourselves responsibly before God—*solus cum solo*[6]—Father Fuchs states that the notion that "the human person is illuminated by a light that comes, not from one's own reason…but from the wisdom of God in whom everything is created…cannot stand up to an objective analysis nor prove helpful in the vocabulary of Christian believers."[7] Father Fuchs' rejection of the Council's teaching on the nature of conscience at least has the virtue of consistency. It follows from this own doctrine that while God creates, he does not govern the human mind. The human mind is a merely natural light, to which there corresponds a merely natural jurisdiction over ethics. In this way, Fuchs and other moral theologians have made it clear that the current debate is not merely an in-house controversy between different schools of ethics. The debate reaches the ground of the possibility of any moral theology. The Pope clearly understands the seriousness of the challenge.

Turning to the injunction in Gn. 2.17, the Pope writes: "By forbidding man to 'eat of the tree of the knowledge of good and evil,' God makes it clear that man does not originally possess such 'knowledge' as something properly his own, but only participates in it by the light of natural reason and of Divine Revelation, which manifest to him the requirements and promptings of eternal wisdom. Law must therefore be considered an expression of divine wisdom…" (no. 41). The natural condition of man is one of participation in a higher norm. Man has liberty to direct himself because he is first directed by another.[8]

The Pope makes use of a number of authorities to express the idea of natural law as "participated theonomy."[9] He refers to Ps. 4.6, "Let the light of your face shine upon us, O Lord," emphasizing that moral knowledge derives from a divine illumination;[10] from Rom. 2.14, "The Gentiles who had not the Law, did naturally the things of the Law," he calls attention to the idea that it is not just by positive law that humans are directed in the moral order;[11] from Gregory of Nyssa, he cites the passage that autonomy is predicated only of a king;[12] from St. Bonaventure, he cites the dictum that conscience does not bind on its own authority, but is rather the "herald of a king" (no. 58). The very existence of conscience, the Pope argues, indicates that we are under a law that we did not impose upon ourselves.[13] Conscience is not a witness to a human power; it is a witness to the natural law. And this is only to say that the natural law is a real law which cannot be equated with our conscience. It was precisely this equation, the pope notes, that beguiled our first parents, when the serpent in Gn. 3.5 said they could be as gods. What does it mean to be as gods? It means that the human mind is a measuring-measure, having authority to impart the measures of moral good and evil.[14]

If there is anything in moral theology on which the Fathers held a unanimous opinion it was that the injunction in Genesis 2.17 summarizes the natural law. As early as the 2nd century, Tertullian characterized this injunction "as the womb of all the precepts of God"—a "law unwritten, which was habitually understood naturally."[15] Law did not begin with the law of the Jewish state; though the decalogue is a divine positive law, it reiterates (in the relation between the two tables) the original ordering reported in Genesis. There never was a sphere of lawless ethics; that is to say, a sphere in which the created mind posits moral norms without any antecedent rule of law. God governed men from the very outset. Indeed, the idea that there is a lawless morality, possessed by men as a kind of natural right, is precisely the sin committed by our first parents. The first law establishes the rule of law itself, which is that men govern only by sharing in divine governance.

Throughout the scriptures, this rule of law is reitererated. We can have rectitude in matters of ethics only insofar as the mind adheres to God (first by natural law, then through the Law, and finally through grace). Thus, in Mk. 12.28, we read: "And one of the scribes…asked him, 'Which commandment is the first of all?' Jesus answered [quoting Deut 6.4], 'The first is, 'Hear O Israel: The Lord our God, the Lord is one; and you shall love the Lord your God with all your heart, and with all your soul, and with all your mind, and with all your strength.' The second is this 'You shall love your neighbor as yourself.'"

In his commentary on Genesis against the Manicheans, Augustine insisted that the sin of our first parents was a violation of the very core of the natural law. "This is what they were persuaded to do; to love to excess their own power. And since they wanted to be equal to God, they used wrongly, that is, against the Law of God, that middle rank by which they were subject to God and held their bodies in subjection. This middle rank was like the fruit of the tree placed in the middle of paradise. Thus they lost what they had received in wanting to seize what they had not received. For the nature of man did not receive the capability of being happy by its own power without God ruling it. Only God can be happy by his own power with no one ruling."[16]

And the very last of the Fathers, St. Bernard, in his sermons on the Canticle of Canticles, referred to the field in Genesis 2: "He claims our earth not as his fief but as his motherland. And why not? He receives from it his Bride and his very body…as Lord he rules over it; as Creator, he controls it; as Bridegroom, he shares it."[17] God has dominion over the vineyard, and it is by participating in that dominion that human beings are properly ordered. Given this rule, God goes on to make us shareholders in a more profound way, through a wedding. The mystery hidden for the ages in God is that the human participation in divine governance through law was but a preparation for a wedding feast."

By organizing his discussion of natural law around the injunction in Genesis 2.17, the Pope might seem to be indulging a rather abstract meditation. But this is the bottom line. The Pope understands very clearly that the contemporary dispute over law and liberty is not a dispute merely over this or that vexed issue; what is really at stake today is the effort to claim theological warrant for a principle that is essentially anti-theological: viz., the principle that the human mind has a justifiable claim of jurisdiction over the vineyard. This is why the Church cannot make people happy by loosening the law over this or that area of conduct. A loosened law is not what men crave. They want jurisdiction; not liberty, but plenary authority. This anti-theology is at the heart of that curious phenomenon I mentioned earlier. When theologians, clergy, and laity make the plea for authority to be used to annul the law, and in effect to cancel out authority itself, what they are really requesting (even if they do not state it in crisp and unambiguous terms) is for you to hand back authority which they believe is rightfully theirs. This is why the disputes today over moral theology are so nasty.[18] They resemble nothing so much as ruthless litigation over real estate.

III.

Indeed, real estate is the favorite scriptural metaphor for the problem. The request for dominion rather than convenantal participation, along with the illusion that God is an absentee landlord, is the oldest story on the books. This desire for absolute jurisdictional authority amounts to the same story every time. Consider, for example, the parable of the wicked tenants, which is told in each of the synoptic gospels. In Mt. 21, it is told just before the parable of the marriage feast; in Mk. 12, it is given just after the chief priests and the scribes ask Jesus by whose authority he teaches; and in Lk. 20, it is given once again just after Jesus' credentials are questioned.

In Mk. 12.1ff., the parable is told in this way:

> A certain man planted a vineyard and made a hedge around it and dug a place for the winevat and built a tower and let it to tenants; and went into a far country. And at the season he sent to the tenants a servant to receive of them the fruit of the vineyard. Who, having laid hands on him, beat him and sent him away empty. And again he sent to them another servant; and him they wounded in the head and used him reproachfully. And again he sent another and him they killed; and many

others, of whom some they beat, and others they killed. Therefore, having yet one son, most dear to him, he also sent him unto them last of all, saying: They will reverence my son. But the tenants said to one another: this is the heir. Come let us kill him and the inheritance will be ours. And, laying hold of him, they killed him and cast him out of the vineyard. What therefore will the Lord of the vineyard do? He will come and destroy those tenants and will give the vineyard to others.

This parable is often associated with the canticle of the vineyard in Is. 5. Every Jew of course knew by heart the song of Isaiah: "Let me sing to my friend the song of his love for his vineyard. My friend had a vineyard on a fertile hillside. He dug the soil, cleared it of stones, and planted choice vines in it." But let us consider the parable in connection with the story of that earlier vineyard in Genesis 2–3.

Just as in Gn. 2, where God plants and irrigates the plantation, and in Isaiah 5, where God is said to have established Israel as a vineyard, in Mk 12, once again, it is the owner who plants and establishes the field. The parable makes it clear that he has the strong claim to ownership—*dominium* not a mere *ius*. We notice an important difference between the original plantation and the one in the parable. Adam and Eve were given a most attractive lease over the garden: in exchange for minimal upkeep, they were entitled to enjoy all of its pleasures—provided that they not usurp ownership. This deal or proto-covenant is symbolized by the two trees. Whereas in Gn. 2 the plantation is perfect, in the parable the vineyard is new and untried. The tenants in this parable will have to work. It is a post-Edenic situation.

According to Jewish law, a new vineyard was not recognized as profitable until four whole harvests. The produce of the fourth year are legally "first fruits." Prior to the year of first fruits, tenants perhaps were entitled to a fixed proportion of the produce, usually along with some rent. Now, the servant is sent to take the rent. As the parable relates, the tenants beat him and sent him away empty. In ancient Semitic law, giving up of a garment, or the casting off of a shoe, legally signifies releasing a right or a claim. The question is, a right to what? Perhaps the tenants are at first only driving a hard bargain. Until the vineyard is shown to be fruitful, the tenants do not want to pay more than their fair share in a still risky project. Unfortunately, the rights claim seems to escalate.

It was typical in Jewish law that when a thing happens three times it is presumed to be normal. For three successive harvests, no rent was paid: hence a precedent is about to be set. The owner has to come back, lest he forfeit his ownership. In other words, what began as a hard bargain—rights to less rent—ends in a claim over the entire farm. It ends, in fact, in a plot to usurp dominion. They kill the heir. Adam stole dominion, and ruined the original partnership; but things have gotten much nastier in the meantime. Adam merely hid—later, his progeny will be more aggressive. Expelled from the garden, and cast into the world, his progeny now figure that they have a more or less permanent lease, with no strings attached. We should not overlook the fact that the scribes and Pharisees are the object of the parable. Although the prophets warned about this, the scribes and Pharisees believed that God had given them the vineyard, and had left it to them to call the shots. The Scribes and Pharisees were like Deists; they dug in their heels for the long haul. Everything is fine so long as He doesn't come back. And when the Lord of the vineyard returned, they killed him.

IV

The meaning of the parable for moral theology ought to be clear. Moral theologians must not be lawyers for the tenants. The Pope writes in *Veritatis Splendor*:

> Even if moral-theological reflection usually distinguishes between the positive or revealed law of God and the natural law, and, within the economy of salvation, between the "old" and the "new" law, it must not be forgotten that these and other useful distinctions always refer to that law whose author is the one and the same God and which is always meant for man. The different ways in which God, acting in history, cares for the world and for mankind are not mutually exclusive; on the contrary, they support each other and intersect.... God's plan poses no threat to man's genuine freedom; on the contrary, the acceptance of God's plan is the only way to affirm that freedom. (VS no. 45)

Beginning in Genesis 2, and then with the election of Israel, and continuing with the establishment of the Church, and ending in Revelation 22, where the vineyard finally is transfigured by the Tree of Life, God asserts authority over the field. Father De Lubac points out that although God makes "fresh starts in his work and devises fresh methods to bring it to a successful conclusion, it is by no means a fresh work that he undertakes."[20] Even if, according to the parable of the treasure hidden in the field, God eventually had to stop negotiating and buy back the property, repurchasing it with the blood of his own Son, at each stage in this history God offers something covenantal to the tenants. God always makes participation the terms of the deal; men always want unilateral authority.

At every stage, the lease included ample scope for the liberty and creativity of the tenants. Our first parents could eat of every tree but one; they were permitted to name the beasts. They were not permitted, however, to claim absolute dominion. Why? Because what is at stake in the covenant, including that proto-covenant with created nature in Genesis 2, is not merely a deal regarding the administration of external properties. These things were always meant for man. Over them man always had enormous freedom. What was at stake was something internal, the order of justice according to which men act in communion with God.[21] But we cannot act in communion with God if we unilaterally claim the law for ourselves. Again, the prophets warned the rabbinical establishment not to make the Law a mere interpretive tool to be used for their own convenience. And we must admit that this story of the wicked tenants, and the lessons to be drawn from it, is relevant to the life of the Church, and will continue to be relevant until the final reconciliation.

C. S. Lewis urges us to recall the parable of the prodigal, which reiterates the story of Genesis. "As a young man wants a regular allowance from his father which he can count on as his own, within which he makes his own plans (and rightly, for his father is a fellow creature) so they desired to be on their own, to take care for their own future, to plan for pleasure and for security, to have a *meum* from which, no doubt, they would pay some reasonable tribute to God in the way of time, attention, and love, but which nevertheless, was theirs not His. They wanted, as we say, to 'call their souls their own.' But that means to live a lie, for our souls are not, in fact, our own. They wanted some corner for the universe of which they could say to God, 'This is our business, not yours...'"

As the Pope notes at the outset of *Veritatis,* a "new situation" has come about. Opposition, even within the seminaries, to Catholic moral doctrine is "no longer a matter of limited and occasional dissent, but of an overall and systematic calling into question of traditional moral doctrine" (VS no. 4). Whenever we see men demand that authority be used to subvert authority, and that law be used to annul the law, we know that we are close to the heart of the story. Rights claims escalate into a claim over the entire farm.

The message for moral theologians is that they must never pervert their craft by being lawyers for the tenants against the Lord. When they act like lawyers for the tenants, they play the role of the Scribes and Pharisees, who also wanted to call the shots by turning the law into their own interpretive tool. Whereas the Scribes and Pharisees laid hold of the positive law, twisting it to their own purposes, our moral theologians are more tempted to use the rubric of natural law. The Pope, however, is not going to turn the farm over to the tenants. The farm does not belong to him. The moral theologians insist that he must. Indeed, they threaten to take it anyway. But we already know how this story must end.

Notes

1. Regrettably, the NCCB evinces this attitude in its advertisement for *Veritatis Splendor*: "It reverses pre-Vatican II legalism by speaking of the good and the bad rather than the forbidden and permitted, and by speaking about the invitation to live a moral life in God rather than the enforcing of laws or norms." This characterization is in tune with the *New York Times*, whose recent Sunday Magazine article on the Pope (12/11/94) summarized the question before the next pope: "More law, or more love?"

2. Josef Fuchs, *Moral Demands and Personal Obligations*, trans. Brian McNeil (Washington, D.C.: Georgetown University Press, 1993), 100.

3. Id., 55. Concerning "the various persons who have been given the requisite intellectual capacity," one suspects that Father Fuchs has in mind the ersatz magisterium of moral theologians.

4. Janet Smith, *Humanae Vitae: A Generation Later* (Washington, D.C.: The Catholic University Press of America, 1991), 23.

5. Fuchs, 39.

6. "Deep within his conscience man discovers a law which he has not laid upon himself but which he must obey. Its voice, ever calling him to love and to do what is good and to avoid evil, tells him inwardly at the right moment: do this, shun that. For man has in his heart a law inscribed by God. His dignity lies in observing this law, and by it he will be judged. His conscience is man's most secret core, and

his sanctuary. There he is alone with God whose voice echoes in his depths" (GS, n. 16).

7. Fuchs, 157.

8. In scholastic parlance, the human reason is a measuring measure (*mensura mensurans*) only insofar as it is first a measured measure (*mensura mensurata*).

9. "Others speak, and rightly so, of theonomy, or participated theonomy, since man's free obedience to God's law effectively implies that human reason and human will participate in God's wisdom and providence" (VS no. 41).

10. VS, no. 2.

11. VS, nos. 12, 46.

12. VS, no. 38.

13. "The judgment of conscience does not establish the law; rather it bears witness to the authority of the natural law and of the practical reason with reference to the supreme good, whose attractiveness the human person perceives and whose commandments he accepts" (no. 60).

14. "Were this autonomy to imply a denial of the participation of the practical reason in the wisdom of the divine Creator and Lawgiver, or were it to suggest a freedom which creates moral norms, on the basis of historical contingencies or the diversity of societies and cultures, this sort of alleged autonomy would contradict the Church's teaching on the truth about man. It would be the death of true freedom: 'But of the tree of the knowledge of good and evil you shall not eat, for in the day that you eat of it you shall die' (Gn 2:17)" (VS, no. 40).

15. "quasi matrix praeceptorum Dei...non scriptam, quae naturaliter intelligebatur" *Adv. Judaeos*, cap. 2 (PL 2-2, 599, 600).

16. *De Genesi contra Manichaeos*, II cap. 9, no. 12. The same point is made in VS, nos. 54-55.

17. *Sermones super cantica canticorum*, Sermon 59, I.2.

18. In the *London Tablet* Bernard Haring recently rejected the papal encyclical *Veritatis Splendor,* basing his objection (in part) on a right of conscience grounded in natural law. See *National Catholic Reporter* (Nov. 5, 1993).

19. For a shrewd analysis of this parable, see J. Duncan M. Derrett, *Law in the New Testament* (London: Darton, Longman & Todd, 1970). From Derrett I have learned not only the connection between the parable in Mk 12 and Gn 2, but also some of the details of ancient Semitic law which form the background of the parable.

20. Henri de Lubac, *Catholicism: Christ and the Common Destiny of Man.* English translation of *Catholicisme*, (Paris: Editions du Cerf, 1947) by Lancelot C. Sheppard and Sister Elizabeth Englund (San Francisco: Ignatius, 1988), 261f.

21. "For 'a religious man' means not so much 'one who is capable of religious experiences' (as is generally supposed) as above all 'one who is just to God the Creator'" Karol Wojtyla, *Love and Responsibility*, trans. H. T. Willetts (San Francisco: Ignatius Press, 1981), 223.

22. C. S. Lewis, *The Problem of Pain* (New York: MacMillan Pub., 1962), 80.

23. As St. Bernard remarks: "is it not all God's farm, God's building, the vineyard of the Lord of Sabbaoth?" (*Sermones super cantica canticorum*, Sermon no. 63, II.3). It should be noted that Bernard is here referring to the "little foxes" who destroy the vines of the vineyard.

Chapter 3

MORAL ABSOLUTES
IN THE CIVILIZATION OF LOVE

The Reverend Romanus Cessario, O.P.

As an authentic expression of magisterial teaching, the encyclical *Veritatis Splendor* enunciates Christian truth for God's people who live within the economy of faith.[1] Still, as many commentators have observed, the present encyclical also represents a new initiative in the history of magisterial teaching. The Magisterium of course has addressed "the sphere of morals" and has even taught "specific particular precepts" throughout the course of the Church's history.[2] But because *Veritatis Splendor* undertakes to expound "fundamental questions of the Church's moral teaching," it provides authoritative norms for establishing the morality of all kinds of human actions.[3] In other words, the encyclical takes up the challenge of helping each believer to answer, what the Holy Father calls, "the primordial question": What is good and evil? What must be done to have eternal life? (no. 111).

An episode in the life of St. Thomas's commentator, Cardinal Cajetan, illustrates both the nature and the difficulty of the challenge that Pope John Paul II engaged in writing this encyclical. In the sixteenth century, Cajetan advanced the view that the personal condition of an agent should figure in the moral evaluation of his or her actions. But because Cajetan's effort to discuss morality from "the perspective of the acting person" was premature, it earned him a reputation, even among some of his fellow Dominicans, for promoting moral laxism—a high misdemeanor during this period of nascent casuistry. Why this reaction? Cajetan's opponents reasoned thusly: to hold that an adequate moral evaluation of an action must take account of its "object" as "*rationally chosen by the deliberate will*"—to borrow an important phrase from the encyclical (see no. 78)—means considering the psychological condition of the person who makes a moral choice. This in turn leads to making subjective excuses for violations of the moral law. Cajetan, of course, was neither a laxist nor a revisionist *ante nomen*. He was simply applying what Aquinas had developed theologically from Aristotle's *Nicomachean Ethics*. Aquinas speaks about the nature of moral science—namely, it concerns practical knowledge. Unlike theoretical knowledge which informs the mind with specific truths, practical knowledge is ordered ultimately to what a person either makes or does. For this reason, practical knowledge depends on the character of the one who possesses it in a way that speculative knowledge does not. To give a concrete example, a person can engage in bad actions and still function as a good mathematician. However, no one should expect to receive good advice about sobriety from a person who habitually drinks too much.[4]

In continuity with the teaching of the Apostles, *Veritatis Splendor* talks about practical knowledge; specifically, it concerns "*the right conduct of Christians*" (no. 26). As an exercise in practical knowledge, Christian moral theology includes accounts of the "good," the commandments, the virtues, the gifts of the Holy Spirit and the Beatitudes as well as of moral judgments, e.g., "It is good to help others in distress," at whatever level of generality such judgments are expressed. But unlike geometry, which can draw a true conclusion from its own theoretical principles, moral science ensures completely practical knowledge, the knowledge incarnate in action, only up to a certain point.[5] Why? Completely practical knowledge requires moral agency, and choice always implies the exercise of human freedom. On the basis of this analysis, we might speculate that Cajetan's opponents regarded moral teaching to be more like geometry than in fact is the case: the important thing is to get the [moral] theorem right. Cajetan, on the other hand, understood that it is one thing to affirm the orthodox doctrine on the Trinity, and another to affirm the moral truth that "it is good to help others in distress." When the Christian believes the orthodox doctrine of the Trinity, he or she can be said to possess the truth in faith, whereas when the believer learns that "it is good to help others in distress," he or she still needs to move to the moment of completely practical knowledge, to render the knowledge incarnate in action. In other words, the believer must choose the good and, influenced by the virtue of prudence, command the good action.

To recognize the way that moral truth informs prudence is not to deny the value of moral science, together with its postulates and arguments, for the Christian life. Moral norms are important, and the Pastors of the Church must proclaim them as constitutive elements of the Church's call to conversion. A lesson from history illustrates the importance of sound teaching. In her study of women, the family and Nazi politics entitled *Mothers in the Fatherland*, Claudia Koonz discovered that during the period of the National Socialist Party in Germany women reacted no differently than men when it came to opposing unjust laws. The only exception were Roman Catholic nurses, who, because they had been taught that sterilization was wrong, objected to its inclusion in the health care directives of the Third Reich. Normative instruction, then, is important. Even so, *Veritatis Splendor* invites us to look at the moral life from the point of view of the acting person. So in this paper, I would like to argue that a specific strength of the encyclical lies in its presentation of the moral life as situated within the larger context of the theological life. While the Holy Father touches many aspects of the Christian moral life, I develop three of these: the connaturality of virtue, especially prudence; freedom in Christ; and the happy life, what the classical authors call beatitude.

*   *   *

Today Cajetan is not much remembered as a moralist. While his commentaries on the *Summa Theologiae* inspired a great deal of philosophy and dogmatic theology during the period of the twentieth-century Leonine revival, Cajetan's teaching on morals, even his important commentaries on prudence, remained relatively unknown.[6] Instead, the sixteenth century witnessed the development of legalistic casuistry, which eclipsed the classical moral teaching on the virtues. By developing treatises on the virtues, the ancient Christian authors concretized the graced connaturality between man and the true good.[7] The casuist systems controlled the moral context of the Church for roughly four centuries, from the mid-sixteenth century through the first half of the twentieth century.[8] In my view, many of the difficulties that moral theology has suffered over the past thirty years, and which *Veritatis Splendor* addresses, derive in large measure from the fact that one of the least publicized events that took place at the Second Vatican Council was the bringing of a four hundred year-old casuist tradition to closure. *Veritatis Splendor* indeed introduces a new era in the history of moral theology. Certain of my fellow Catholic moral theologians interpret the significance of the encyclical differently. Some claim that the text should be read as mere exhortation, a "papal *cri de coeur*,"[9] whereas others predict that its influence will be short-lived.[10] I am not persuaded by these dismissive arguments. Why? Because, as Alasdair MacIntyre's analysis of the encyclical points out, *Veritatis Splendor* presents us "with what is in effect a theology of moral philosophy embedded in a theology of the moral life."[11] Except for a truncated account of the four last things, death, judgment, heaven, and hell, the casuist theologians offered the Church no theology of the moral life.

Again, *Veritatis Splendor* signals a new beginning for moral theology. In an unambiguously clear way, the encyclical sets forth the need for "exceptionless moral norms" (no. 82), but without recapitulating the rigid legalism and confusion of the old casuistry. In other words, we should not expect that post-*Veritatis Splendor* moral theology will produce a new collection of moral manuals, complete with detailed lists of moral precepts and instructions for resolving "cases of conscience" in a way that mimics legal jurisprudence. Rather, the moral theology of the new evangelization aims to develop first a communion of persons (*communio personarum*) in which individuals are shaped by the truth of the divine and evangelical law. Among other benefits of the new personalism, Pastors of the Church can speak confidently even about the "*universality and immutability*" of the natural law because they know, with St. Augustine, that these norms reflect divine truth.[12] The Holy Father makes an especially bold claim: "*this universality does not ignore the individuality of human beings,* nor is it opposed to the absolute uniqueness of each person. On the contrary, it embraces at its root each of the person's free acts, which are meant to bear witness to the universality of the true good" (no. 51). This means that *Veritatis Splendor* requires us to think now in terms of a virtue-centered approach to moral theology, one that relies on the cardinal virtue of prudence, as much as on the canons of moral jurisprudence. The better that moral theologians work out the principles set down in the encyclical, the more easily the Church will be able to show that "man's *genuine moral autonomy* in no way means the rejection but rather the acceptance of the moral law, of God's command… " (no. 41). Consequently, the prudent man or woman is able to embrace the complete truth-value of Catholic moral teaching, and at the same time exercise a full measure of personal freedom. In the technical language of the encyclical, this state is described as one of "theonomy" or of "participated theonomy."[13] In short, Pope John Paul calls us to a vertical transcendence, which is at the source of every love, and which alone can perfect the spiritual nature of the human person.[14] Aquinas captures the same truth when he says, "God alone satisfies."[15]

It is not surprising, then, that the Holy Father makes a central point of Thomist moral theology his own: "It is the 'heart' converted to the Lord and to the love of what is good which is really the source of *true* judgments of conscience. Indeed, in order to 'prove what is the will of God, what is good and acceptable and perfect' (Rom 12: 2), knowledge of God's law in general is certainly necessary, but it is not sufficient: what is essential is a sort of '*connaturality' between man and the true good.*"[16] As Martin Rhonheimer points out, only this kind of virtuous connaturality enables a person to develop "the genuine perspective of morals," which, Rhonheimer argues, is one of the truly innovative parts of the encyclical's teaching about moral objects.[17] The moral condition of the person affects the judgment of prudence.

Upright living supports prudence, whereas vicious habits impair, and can even destroy, a person's capacity to realize completely practical knowledge in accord with moral truth. The Holy Father reserves the term freedom to characterize the person who not only knows what the moral law teaches, but who also is able to render moral truth incarnate in his or her actions.

* * *

So we come to another feature of the theology of the moral life found in *Veritatis Splendor*, the notion of freedom. Pope John Paul II has accomplished what Cardinal Cajetan had been unable to achieve. The Pope has elaborated a moral theology that places the individual person and personal freedom at the center of moral analysis. He expresses his understanding of the relation between freedom, truth, and the human person, but he does so without endorsing the moral subjectivism that Cajetan's "conservative" adversaries feared in the sixteenth century. Of course, neither does he countenance the moral waffling which many neo-casuists in the twentieth century consider inescapable. The success of Pope John Paul in setting forth a teaching that both upholds moral truth and takes full account of human freedom is due, at least in part, to his acquaintance with modern philosophy, especially modern theories of ethics and anthropology.

In *The Acting Person,* John Paul II took the characteristically modern notions of self-possession, self-determination, and self-governance and placed them within the biblical context of conditional stewardship and respect for the divine sovereignty. As Kenneth Schmitz has explained in his illuminating work, *At the Center of the Human Drama,* Karol Wojtyla a was uniquely prepared to talk from the Chair of Peter about the absolute character of moral truth, while at the same time affirming that human freedom forms part of "the ontological structure of man."[18] "It seems to me," writes Schmitz, "that to John Paul II's mind the modern practical tendency to obscure or forget the conditional nature of our stewardship is the direct outcome of the modern theoretical tendency to treat human consciousness as an absolute."[19] The ethics of health care, for example, requires a renewed commitment to conditional stewardship, including the stewardship of one's own physical life. Moral absolutes represent one way of concretizing the requirements of this conditional stewardship, so that the enthusiasm generated by technological developments, which has shaped the modern mind since the seventeenth century, will not frustrate the development of the civilization of love.

It would be misleading, however, to suggest that the Pope's acquaintance with modern philosophical categories alone enables him to supply a moral teaching that takes account of human freedom and at the same time re-affirms the universal validity of the negative precepts of the natural law, which "oblige each and every individual, always and in every circumstance" (no. 52). For the Church could not adequately account for the place that human freedom holds in the Christian life, unless she had also determined the nature of Christ's human freedom. Recall that the encyclical gives us a "theology of the moral life." This theology of the moral life owes much to the sixth ecumenical council, III Constantinople (681), which rejected the monothelitist heresy (*DS* 556). It is illustrative to reflect on the fact that the "monophysitic mentality" about Christ perdured for more than two centuries after the Council of Chalcedon (451). In this view of the Incarnation lurks the conviction that human freedom disappears in the presence of divine grace. In other words, no human action or genuine human autonomy remains once a divine action has begun to work in a person. As pious as this explanation may appear, it in fact destroys the Christian view of man and empties the expression "participated theonomy" of any meaning. Rather, the biblical doctrine on creation obliges us to accept that human actions have a value in their own right: God created man a unity of body and soul—*corpore et anima unus.*[20] What is more to the point, the first person to demonstrate that human actions can possess divine value is Christ himself. So the Pope can affirm that "human freedom and God's law are not in opposition; on the contrary, they appeal one to the other" (no. 17). In the person of Jesus Christ, the Church beholds the "concrete norm"—to borrow a phrase from von Balthasar—of human freedom and divine law appealing one to the other. This "concrete norm," moreover, is not a luxury for the human race, as if believers enjoy a slightly better position than non-believers do when it comes to distinguishing right from wrong. For as the "concrete norm" of the moral life, Christ himself alone makes it possible for the human person to achieve his or her most high calling through the exercise of both the theological virtues and the infused moral virtues.[21]

"Christ the new Adam, in the very revelation of the mystery of the Father and of his love, fully reveals man to himself and brings to light his most high calling."[22] This cardinal principle of post-conciliar theology is put to new use in the encyclical: The Pope reminds us that only the Lord bestows on us the full enabling condition of freedom. The scholastic discussions about the relative sufficiency of the acquired virtues addressed this same issue in pre-modern categories. Allow me to return to Cajetan for a moment. As a Christian humanist, Cajetan was willing to grant that, since the acquired virtues are true virtues, they could establish a relative perfection (what he termed the "essence of virtue"). But he also held that the acquired virtues by themselves could not produce what he called the state of virtue, the full "status virtutis." For only charity orders the virtues to the Ultimate End in an unqualified fashion. If we follow Cajetan's view on the relative sufficiency of the human virtues, then we must conclude that before the salvific life and death of the God-man, human autonomy could not even achieve the ultimate good of the very nature that it served. For only the charity of Christ makes the virtues of human life exist in full existential possession of their efficacy. This is the first principle of the theology of the moral life that provides the matrix for the encyclical's specific moral teaching. Just as Christ, because he remains the Eternal Word of Truth, exercises his authentic human freedom in a way that always embodies the greatest charity or love, so the one who remains united to Christ enjoys the assurance that his or her actions embody the full measure of moral truth.

In Chapter Three of *Veritatis Splendor*, entitled "Lest the Cross of Christ Be Emptied of its Power" (1 Cor 1:17), the Pope urges the Church, and especially her priests, to undertake "an intense pastoral effort," so that the "essential bond between Truth, the Good and Freedom" will be better known in the world (see no. 84). If the Church is to avoid endorsing the measures of expediency that are so seductive to the modern spirit, each member of the Church must be completely persuaded of this fundamental Christian truth, namely, "when all is said and done, the law of God is always the one true good of man" (ibid.).[23] To avoid raising expediency to the level of a moral principle, however, we cannot remain only at the side of Christ the Divine

Teacher. We must also be ready to stand by the Cross of the Crucified Christ; in other terms, we must become disciples of the Cross. It is incumbent on the Pastors of the Church to show that this vocation does not go against the good of reason. They need to affirm unequivocally that the wisdom of the Cross creates neither foolishness nor stumbling block (see 1 Cor 23). Rather, to circumvent the wisdom of the Cross means inviting death-dealing disobedience. St. Irenaeus writes: "The Lord, coming into his own creation in visible form, was sustained by his own creation which he himself sustains in being. His obedience on the tree of the cross reversed the disobedience at the tree in Eden."[24] Aquinas teaches the same truth when he explains the true purpose of the Incarnation. While the end or objective of the Incarnation entails the perfection of our godly image, the motive for the Incarnation remains the fact that a disobedient people required a Savior to reverse their lot. An essential feature of the ministry of the moral theologian is to help people acknowledge their sins, so that Christian believers can move beyond the stage of image-restoration, which entails sorrow and conversion, to that of image-perfection, which is the state of genuine freedom. In fact, the Pope states that "*The Crucified Christ reveals the authentic meaning of freedom; he lives it fully in the total gift of himself* and calls his disciples to share in his freedom" (no. 85).

    Veritatis Splendor is really a soteriological document, for it urges us to confront the false voices of freedom that cry out in "many different 'areopagi'."[25] Given the secularization of the West, these voices are numerous, heard especially in the areopagus of social welfare agencies as well as that of health-care professionals. For this reason, special discernment is required in these fields in order to distinguish the "authentic meaning of freedom," a freedom which always leads to excellence, from freedom which is false because it is not "in harmony with the true good of the person" (no. 72). The true good of the person can never be compromised for reasons of expediency. For even one bad choice, so the Holy Father affirms, puts "us in conflict with our ultimate end, the supreme good, God himself" (ibid.).

* * *

If freedom is the distinctive feature of ethical action, practical action only reaches completion in the good. When discussing the nature of human action, the *Catechism of the Catholic Church,* Part Three, Section One, generally follows the outline of Aquinas's *prima secundae.* The *Catechism* treats first our vocation to beatitude (1716-1729), next human freedom (1730-1742), and then the virtues and gifts of the Holy Spirit (1803-1832) which account for our personal transformation as well as our free participation in beatitude. (It is significant that Aquinas retained the patristic view that the virtues and the gifts remain with the saints in heaven, even though they no longer face moral choices.) In order to stress the order of development in the human person, I have in this paper reversed the order of presentation, namely, virtue, freedom, beatitude. This also allows me, while discussing Christian happiness, to refer more explicitly to the important question of health care issues. Today, health care ethics poses one of the strongest challenge to the observance of moral absolutes. For even at its highest level, the human good must include provision for sustaining the physiological and biological level of human nature. As Pope John Paul has had occasion to teach repeatedly, the failure to respect human life from the moment of conception to natural death devastates the civilization of love.

Let me introduce the general issue of health care in light of the three points that I am making in this paper. *Veritatis Splendor* affirms the significance of the "objective moral order" for bringing about true Christian personalism.[26] Many of our contemporaries are persuaded that individual conditions, especially those which surround difficult health care situations, make it nearly impossible to apply general moral principles or "to establish any particular norm the content of which would be binding without exception" (no. 82). I have argued, however, that the variables associated with caring for the sick and dying should urge Christian believers to rely on the virtue of prudence. This means that having been shown "the inviting splendor of that truth which is Jesus Christ himself" (no. 83), their minds will be conformed to the full moral truth about human life. While it is true that only the prudent person acts virtuously in a particular circumstance, the Church—as *Donum Vitae* reminds us—must proclaim to the world that human life is sacred and that God alone is the master of life (see no. 5). So both the 1980 "Declaration on Euthanasia" and the 1974 "Declaration on Procured Abortion" assert, as the latter puts it, that "the first right of the human person is the right to life" (no. 11). *Veritatis Splendor* develops this assertion when it teaches that abstaining from the intentional killing of innocent human life remains, no matter what the circumstances or further intentions, *semper et pro semper* an indispensable condition for attaining Christian happiness. No prudent person can choose to act against this norm: it grounds the drive to happiness.

The encyclical cites St. Augustine's *Commentary on John*: "The beginning of freedom is to be free from crimes…such as murder, adultery, fornication, theft, fraud, sacrilege, and so forth. When once one is without these crimes (and every Christian should be without them), one begins to lift up one's head towards freedom" (no. 13). Thus, Catholic moral teaching on care of the sick and dying aims to ennoble Christian believers, to make them perfectly free, to bring them toward a perfection that is due each human person. The *Catechism of the Catholic Church* recalls that Jesus repeats the commandment, "Thou shalt not kill," during his Sermon on the Mount (see Mt 5:21).[27] This biblical text invites us to consider the context of moral absolutes. The *Ethical and Religious Directives for Catholic Health Care Services* should not be treated as burdensome obligations that Catholics have to endure, but rather they should be accepted as reliable guides to beatitude.[28] A text from St. Augustine, which is not found in the encyclical, helps us understand the importance of making the proper decision in matters of health care: "For in the way you decide to follow Christ, this you have intended, this you have chosen, this is your judgment."[29] Even in seemingly difficult cases, such as assisted suicide, direct sterilization, human embryo research, and the treatment of rape victims, the reason for determining a wise and truthful course of action is to ensure that the Christian believer as well as those who care for him or her attain the positive goal of Christian happiness. As the Christian believer acts under the influence of infused prudence and with the aid of the gift of the Holy Spirit, he or she already possesses the Good. "Genuine freedom is an outstanding manifestation of the divine image in man. For God willed to leave man 'in the power of his own counsel' (see Sir 15:14), so that he would seek his Creator of his own accord and would freely arrive at full and blessed perfection by cleaving to God" (no. 34).[30]

Do we need Catholic health care services? Of course, we do. For the sick and dying should enjoy the same opportunity to continue in the path of blessedness that Catholic moral teaching marks out for them as do those members of the Church who enjoy good health and the prospect of many years. As a Catholic has lived a virtuous life, so he or she has a right to proper health care and, when the Lord comes, to die virtuously, to die choosing Christ. We still refer to this as the grace of a happy death. To die well belongs to the happy life.

In conclusion: *Veritatis Splendor* makes three important contributions to the formation of Catholic health care policy and to the general field of Christian ethics. First, it affirms that since natural law properly "understood does not allow for any division between freedom and nature" (no. 50), we must develop, by nature and in grace, the connaturality of virtue. Second, it explains that since true freedom flows from "communion of life with Christ" (no. 16), it poses no hardship for the believer to accept that "there are certain specific kinds of behavior that are always wrong to choose, because choosing them involves a disorder of the will, that is, a moral evil" (no. 78).[31] Third, in this life, the pursuit of beatitude entails suffering. "Christ's witness is the source, model and means for the witness of his disciples, who are called to walk on the same road: 'If any man would come after me, let him deny himself and take up his cross daily and follow me' (Lk 9: 23)" (no. 89). In my view, these three principles animate the teaching of the encyclical on respect for and proper care of human life.

But we must remember that the New Testament puts us under the sign of the diminutive. The Kingdom grows like the mustard seed; only ideologies look for sudden success. Yet ideologies are destined to fail, whether they appear incarnated in the omnicompetent state or are promulgated in the form of prevailing cultural wisdom. To preach the efficacy of universal and unchanging norms is an invitation to follow the littleness of the beatitudes; it is not a plan for world conquest. And always, the first soul to be converted to this new way of life is our own. The new evangelization begins, then, with each one of us, as we renew our own love of the truth. And this is a grace, one that comes from Christ, reminding us that the Church lives with the sure hope that "all that Christ is we shall become."

Notes

1. "The service to Christian truth which the Magisterium renders is thus for the benefit of the whole People of God called to enter the liberty of the truth revealed by God in Christ" (*Instruction on the Ecclesial Vocation of the Theologian* [1990], no. 14).

2. See no. 110 for the encyclical's explanation as to how the Magisterium properly intervenes in moral theology, which it defines as "a scientific reflection on the *Gospel as the gift and commandment of new life*, a reflection on the life which 'professes the truth in love' (cf. Eph 4:15)." In no. 114, the Holy Father further explains that this task belongs to the threefold *munus, propheticum, sacerdotale,* and *regale* of the priestly office, as set down in the conciliar documents on the Church (*Lumen Gentium)* and on bishops (*Christus Dominus*).

3. The Holy Father himself makes this point: "This is the first time, in fact, that the Magisterium of the Church has set forth in detail the fundamental elements of this [Christian moral] teaching, and presented the principles for the pastoral discernment necessary in practical and cultural situations which are complex and even crucial" (no. 115).

4. Jacques Maritain reflected extensively on the way in which a person's moral character affects his or her moral science. For a discussion of the nuance with which Maritain treats practical knowledge, see Ralph McInerny, *Art and Prudence* (Notre Dame: University of Notre Dame Press, 1988), especially chapter 5, "The Degrees of Practical Knowledge," pp. 63-136.

5. See Ralph McInerny, *Ethica Thomistica* (Washington, D.C.: The Catholic University of America Press, 1982), 38-40.

6. For a treatment of Cajetan's views on moral theology, see Joseph Mayer, "Cajetan comme moraliste," *Revue Thomiste* 39 (1934-35): 343-357.

7. For a thorough study of this theme in the history of moral theology, see Servais Pinckaers, O.P., *The Sources of Christian Ethics,* trans. Sr. Mary Thomas Noble, O.P. (Washington, D.C.: The Catholic University Press of America, 1995).

8. Casuist moral theology divided human actions into two categories: on the one hand, those actions controlled by law, either as enjoined or as forbidden, and, secondly, those actions for which no rule was applicable. These latter, the so-called "free" actions, occurred only because no existing law applied to them. Thus, casuistry placed "free" actions in a secondary place within the moral life. And, in fact, they occurred principally in the areas of piety and devotion.

9. See the report of the remarks made by John Boyle and Anne Patrick at the Moral Theology Group of the Catholic Theological Society of America's 1994 meeting in Baltimore in the *Proceedings of the Catholic Theological Society of America* 49 (1994): 200-201.

10. See Richard McCormick's essay in *America* (30 October 1993): "*Veritatis Splendor* at key points attributes to theologians positions that they do not hold. It will, I predict, eventually enjoy a historical status similar to that of *Humani Generis*" (p. 11).

11. Alasdair MacIntyre, "How Can We Learn What *Veritatis Splendor* Has To Teach?," *The Thomist* 58 (1994): 189.

12. See *De Trinitate*, Bk. 14, 15, 21 (*Corpus Christianorum. Series Latina,* vol. 50/A, p. 451) as quoted in *Veritatis Splendor*, no. 51.

13. See no. 41. For background on this notion, see Joseph de Finance, "Autonomie et Théonomie," in *L'Agire Morale*, ed. M. Zalba (Naples: Edizioni Domenicane Italiane, 1974), 239-260.

14. See Kenneth L. Schmitz, *At the Center of the Human Drama: The Philosophical Anthropology of Karol Wojtyla/Pope John Paul II* (Washington, D.C.: The Catholic University of America, 1993), 86 ff. The author explains how this theme appears even in Wojtyla's early dramas, *Radiation of Fatherhood* and *The Jeweler's Shop*.

15. *Expositio in symbolum apostolicum,* 1.

16. *Veritatis Splendor* no. 64, citing *Summa Theologiae* II-II, q. 45, a. 2. Pope Pius XII made a similar point in *Humani Generis* when he affirmed that "never has Christian philosophy denied the usefulness and efficacy of good dispositions of soul for perceiving and embracing moral and religious truths" (no. 34).

17. See Martin Rhonheimer, "'Intrinsically Evil Acts' and the Moral Viewpoint: Clarifying a Central Teaching of *Veritatis Splendor*," *The Thomist* 58 (1994): 1-39. Rhonheimer goes on to point out that a genuine perspective of morals reveals an intimate relation between the "object" and the "will" or "choice," so that the object becomes understood as "the proximate end of a deliberate decision which determines the act of willing..." (*Veritatis Splendor*, no. 78).

18. See Schmitz, *At the Center*, 104.

19. Ibid., 97.

20. The *Catechism* cites an important text from *Gaudium et Spes,* no. 14.1: "Man, though made of body and soul, is a unity. Through his very bodily condition he sums up in himself the elements of the material world. Through him they are thus brought to the highest perfection and can raise their voice in praise freely given to the Creator. For this reason man may not despise his bodily life. Rather he is obliged to regard his body as good and to hold it in honor since God has created it and will raise it up on the last day." The encyclical turns to this text in order to support its refutation of the charge that the traditional concept of natural law entails a physicalism or biologism.

21. See *Gaudium et Spes*, no. 22. See the *Catechism of the Catholic Church*, nos. 1812-1813 for the theological virtues; and nos. 2803 & 2607 for the use of the term "theologal" to describe the life lived according to the theological virtues.

22. Vatican Council II, Pastoral Constitution on the Church in the Modern World, *Gaudium et Spes*, no. 22.

23. This remark is taken from an *Address* to those taking part in the International Congress of Moral Theology (10 April 1986), 2: *Insegnamenti* IX, 1 (1986): 970-71.

24. *Adversus haereses,* Bk. 5, 19, 1 (*Sources chrétiennes,* vol. 153, pp. 248-250).

25. "The more the West is becoming estranged from its Christian roots, the more it is becoming missionary territory, taking the form of many different 'areopagi'" (*Tertio Millennio Adveniente*, no. 57).

26. Citing *Dignitatis Humanae*, no. 7 at *Veritatis Splendor*, no. 82.

27. No. 2262

28. For the full text of these guidelines issued by the Bishops of the United States, see *Origins*, vol. 24: no. 27 (15 December 1994).

29. *Enarationes,* 36, 1, 7 (*Corpus Christianorum. Series Latina,* vol. 38, p. 342).

30. The text cites *Gaudium et Spes,* no. 17.

31. This text is found in the *Catechism of the Catholic Church,* no. 1761.

Chapter 4

UTERINE ISOLATION

The Reverend Germain Kopaczynski, O.F.M., Conv.

Appreciation for Moralists and
Health Care Professionals in the Discussion

When I was in the seminary back in the 60s, a lively discussion arose one day during theology class. (The exchange, if my memory on this matter is correct, was occasioned by Schillebeeckx's *Christ the*

Sacrament of the Encounter with God.) For a while it appeared as if the professor purposely let the debate go on to see where it would lead. Toward the end of the period, as time was winding down, the instructor called on one of my classmates to bring the debate to a close. You will no doubt judge that my classmate was a better theologian than he was a Latin scholar when you hear his answer: "Roma locusta est, causa finita est." Rome is a grasshopper, the case is ended!

As we begin this workshop session on uterine isolation, it is to those whose Latin and theology are more in synch that we owe a debt of gratitude. It is to those theologians and health care professionals whose honesty and integrity kept the issue of uterine isolation alive for several decades and for whom "Roma locuta est" is proper Latin and, more importantly, proper theology that we dedicate this session.

Jesuit Father Thomas O'Donnell is the moralist whose name is most closely associated with the issue of uterine isolation. Indeed, after *Humanae Vitae* was issued in 1968, O'Donnell is practically the only one to continue writing about the procedure.[1] The recent Vatican statement on uterine isolation, written in 1993 and promulgated in 1994, is a precise answer to a precise issue raised by Fr. O'Donnell and several others over what amounts to more than a fifty-year period.[2]

Plausibility of Alternative Positions

"You can't do one thing only." Thus goes the wording of an cardinal tenet of the contemporary ecological movement. In a sense the same proves true in the topic we are discussing. Any attempt to talk about "uterine isolation" alone apart from its historical context will prove illusory. In a sense it is fittingly ironic that we simply cannot isolate uterine isolation from the rest of theology. It will prove to be as true in morality as it is in ecology: you can't do one thing only.

A debate of half a century over what might seem to some a minor point of medical ethics has come to an end for Fr. O'Donnell as we see in his remarks in a recent issue of *Linacre Quarterly*.[3] In it the Jesuit scholar recounts a bit of the history surrounding the 1971-1975 edition of the *Ethical and Religious Directives*. He recalls that a preliminary draft of those *Ethical and Religious Directives*, in dealing with the wider question regarding hysterectomy—remember, you can't do one thing only—contained a statement accepting the validity of tubal ligation under certain very limited conditions.

Father O'Donnell tells us that the genesis of the idea for uterine isolation came about in the course of discussions he had with Dr. Andres Marchetti of Georgetown University Medical Center. Marchetti (a "most solid Catholic" to O'Donnell) spoke of a highly individualized case where the doctor came to two medical judgments:

1. after a cesarean section the uterus could no longer be safely repaired and

2. the patient was not able to withstand the rigors of the hysterectomy at that time.

Marchetti's practice had been to make a repair of the uterus and then go back to do the hysterectomy at another time. Could a simpler procedure be done? Why not *isolate* the uterus from the rest of the system rather than remove it? Hence the birth of the term "uterine isolation."

As the draft of the 1971 *Ethical and Religious Directives* worked its way through the appropriate ethical and ecclesiastical channels, there was a suggestion to revise the wording of Directive 35 of the 1948-1955 *Ethical and Religious Directives* to include the possibility of tubal ligation. A glance at the wording of the Directive 35 of the 1948-1955 *Ethical and Religious Directives* and of the proposed draft of the 1971 directive may prove instructive:

1948-55 ERDs

No. 35: Hysterectomy is not permitted as a routine procedure after any definite number of Caesarean sections. In these cases the pathology of each patient must be considered individually; and care must be had that hysterectomy is not performed as a merely contraceptive measure.

DRAFT PROPOSAL FOR 1971

Hysterectomy is permitted when it is judged to be a necessary means of removing some serious pathology. If in accord with the principle hysterectomy is indicated, the physician may, in accord with his medical judgment, employ the simpler procedure of tubal ligation.

It is with some surprise that we then learn that Father O'Donnell, after seeing the draft proposal and thinking about it, then went about persuading the USCC Dept of Health Affairs to *drop* this version of the directive, especially the reference to "tubal ligation"–after all, it *was* in some ways his brainchild. Why? He tells us that he regarded the reasoning embodied in the notion of tubal ligation "to be only a solidly probable opinion" and as such ought not to appear in the 1971 *Ethical and Religious Directives*.[4] O'Donnell's arguments carried the day. A comparison of the *proposed* 1971 text and the *approved* text may be helpful:

DRAFT PROPOSAL FOR 1971	APPROVED 1971 TEXT
Hysterectomy is permitted when it is judged to be a necessary means of removing some serious pathology. If in accord with the principle hysterectomy is indicated, the physician may, in accord with his medical judgment, employ the simpler procedure of tubal ligation.	**No. 22**: Hysterectomy is permitted when it is sincerely judged to be a necessary means of removing some serious uterine pathological condition. In these cases, the pathological condition of each patient must be considered individually and care must be taken that a hysterectomy is not performed merely as a contraceptive measure, or as a routine procedure after any definite number of Cesarean sections.

Neither the phrase "uterine isolation" nor the more common expression "tubal ligation" has ever appeared in any version of the *Ethical and Religious Directives* approved by the American bishops.

Fr. O'Donnell's 1994 Remarks in *Linacre Quarterly*

In the 1994 *Linacre Quarterly* article to which we referred, Fr. O'Donnell concludes by withdrawing his long-standing view that uterine isolation is a solidly probable opinion which could be followed in practice.[5] In this sense, then, the Jesuit moralist would agree: "Roma locuta est, causa finita est." It may be of some interest to note that Fr. O'Donnell cites an "excellent" article appearing in the January 1993 issue of *Ethics & Medics* which concluded that uterine isolation could not be regarded as an indirect sterilization but rather must be seen as in his words "a directly contraceptive sterilization."[6]

The Question of Sterilization as Seen in the Various Editions of the *Ethical and Religious Directives*

"You can't do one thing only." Fr. O'Donnell has led us to the larger whole of which uterine isolation is but a part, namely, the question of sterilization. It may be helpful to see in schematic form how the *Ethical and Religious Directives* of 1954, 1975, and in 1994 treat the question of sterilization (see opposite page).

The Medical Aspects

During the 1994 Bishops' Workshop, Doctor Thomas Murphy Goodwin spelled out the medical aspects underlying what served as the basis for the theoretical acceptability of uterine isolation in Catholic health care facilities.[7]

"Damaged Uterus"

Goodwin observed that there is no mention in medical literature for the past 30 years of the notion of the "weakened uterus" upon which the theory of uterine isolation is based.[8] Indeed, some ob/gyns suggest that recent evidence leads to the conclusion that, medically speaking, the "weak uterus" simply does not exist.[9] One ob/gyn I consulted told me that he was aware of uterine isolation as a theory about 20 years ago but medical practice since then has made the real-

Sterilization in The Three Versions of the ERDS

1954

No. 31: Procedures that induce sterility, whether permanent or temporary, are permitted when:
a. they are immediately directed to the cure, diminution, or prevention of a serious pathological condition;
b. a simpler treatment is not reasonably available; and
c. the sterility itself is an unintended and, in the circumstances, an unavoidable effect.

No. 35: Hysterectomy is not permitted as a routine procedure after any definite number of Caesarean sections. In these cases the pathology of each patient must be considered individually; and care must be had that hysterectomy is not performed as a merely contraceptive measure.

1975

No. 18: Sterilization, whether permanent or temporary, for men or for women, may not be used as a means of contraception.

No. 20: Procedures that induce sterility, whether permanent or temporary, are permitted when:
a. They are immediately directed to the cure, diminution, or prevention of a serious pathological condition and are not directly contraceptive (that is, contraception is not the purpose); and
b. a simpler treatment is not reasonably available.

No. 22: Hysterectomy is permitted when it is sincerely judged to be a necessary means of removing some serious uterine pathological condition. In these cases, the pathological condition of each patient must be considered individually and care must be taken that a hysterectomy is not performed merely as a contraceptive measure, or as a routine procedure after any definite number of Cesarean sections.

1994

No. 53: Direct sterilization of either men or women, whether permanent or temporary, is not permitted in a Catholic health care institution. Procedures that induce sterility are permitted when their direct effect is the cure or alleviation of a present and serious pathology and a simpler treatment is not available.

ity of "weakened uterus" fade into insignificance, at least in his forty years of ob/gyn experience.

After drawing on studies conducted at Los Angeles County-University of Southern California Women's Hospital from 1983 through 1992, and all the while acknowledging that his is by no means the last word on the topic of uterine isolation, Dr. Goodwin has observed:

> If the ruptured uterus, clearly the most significant type of traumatic uterine injury, can be repaired and the patient allowed to conceive again, how can this or lesser degrees of uterine injury be indications for hysterectomy or 'uterine isolation' in and of themselves? I believe that such data should lead us to revisit the medical-scientific basis for the uterine isolation argument.[10]

Treatment

As a specialist in the field of maternal-fetal medicine, Goodwin is well aware that modern medicine has proven most adept at helping women carry to term pregnancies that not that long ago might have been cause for grave concern. The recent Vatican statement on uterine isolation (1993), far from being unaware of the medical facts, is quite cognizant of recent medical advances in handling difficult pregnancies.[11]

The 1993 Vatican "Responses to Three Questions"

The Language of the Document

I know a priest—a Franciscan interested in ecology, as fate would have it—who speaks of his ardent hope that there be a moratorium on all ecclesiastical pronouncements for a few years to enable us to catch up with our reading, point one, and to keep us from cutting down too many trees, point two. Whatever the merits of this proposal, the 1993 Vatican "Responses to [three] questions proposed concerning 'uterine isolation' and related matters" certainly are brief and to the point. A very quick count comes to 659 words. In this instance, the Congregation is not guilty of verbal or ecological overkill! Three questions, three replies: one affirmative, two negative.

"Sterilization"

As we have come to expect, the Congregation refers us back to previous magisterial statements on the topic of sterilization. "Quaecumque Sterilizatio" of 1975 provides the definition of "direct sterilization" as an action *"whose sole immediate effect is to render the generative faculty incapable of procreation."* Continuing to cite from "Quaecumque," the Congregation adds:

> It [direct sterilization] is absolutely forbidden…according to the teaching of the church, even when it is motivated by a subjectively right intention of curing or preventing a physical or psychological ill effect which is foreseen or feared as a result of pregnancy.

"Direct and Indirect"

Fathers Ford and Kelly in volume two of their *Contemporary Moral Theology* made the very astute observation that one of the major points of disagreement between moralists and medical people is precisely to be found in the importance each group gives to the terms *direct* and *indirect*. To moralists the distinction is crucial; to medical specialists the distinction is often misunderstood. This sage advice will serve us in good stead as we read the Vatican Responses.

In a document of so few words, it is perhaps not without importance to point out that the words "direct" and "indirect" appear seven times in the Responses. In resolving the first case affirmatively, the principle of double effect may be invoked to allow the procedure. Because of the *directly* therapeutic character of the hysterectomy, the sterilization is regarded as *indirect* and hence licit. There is a real medical indication, namely "the curtailing of a serious present danger to the woman independent of a possible future pregnancy."

Different Senses of "Pathology"

There is nothing startling in the use of the language of "direct" and "indirect" for those accustomed to the traditional way the Church handles issues according to the principle of double effect. In point of fact, most of the controversy arising from the Responses hinges around the notion not of "direct" and "indirect" but rather of "pathology."[12] Some attention has also been paid to the temporal dimension that is implied in the use of the word "present" to describe the pathology.[13]

A glance at the medical literature finds that the notion of "pathology" is at once one of the most common as well as one of the most elusive of terms to define. For example, it is discussed everywhere, defined nowhere in the sixteenth edition (1992) of *The Merck Manual of Diagnosis and Therapy*. When "pathology" *is* defined, it is—simply stated—the study of disease. Note the two definitions in *Dorland's Illustrated Medical Dictionary:*

1. That branch of medicine which treats of the essential nature of disease, especially of the structural and functional changes in tissues and organs of the body which cause or are caused by the disease. 2. the structural and functional manifestations of disease.

According to *Butterworths Medical Dictionary*, pathology is defined as: "That branch of medical science that deals with the causes of disease and with their effect on the structure and functions of body tissues." And again as: "The sum of morbid processes and changes that occur in the body tissues in a specified disease."

What do all these medical definitions of "pathology" have in common? An attentive reading provides the answer: Pathology, however wide or narrow it is regarded, deals with *disease.* To understand the reply of the Congregation for the Doctrine of the Faith with respect to uterine isolation, this association of *pathology* with *disease* must be kept in mind.

Regarding the understanding of "pathology," it is perhaps not without significance that *Butterworths* makes the further observation that the term "pathology" has a wider meaning in the United Kingdom than it does in the United States. The last observation might prove especially helpful since in the cases placed before it the Congregation for the Doctrine of the Faith is responding to questions regarding pathology from the United States where, as *Butterworths* notes, "the word [pathology] is confined to morbid anatomical and histopathological studies."[14]

Some press reports which dealt with the Congregation's statement seemed to imply that the Church is overlooking a pathology, a disease, if you will, that is there in some sense.[15] Perhaps this is the key to understanding the precise point of the negative responses given to the second and third questions: the hysterectomy and the uterine isolation are direct sterilizations precisely because THERE IS NO PRESENT PATHOLOGY to speak of. Where there *is* a pathology, such as the one described in the first question, the sterilizations are *indirect* and hence morally allowable; where there *is* no pathology, the sterilizations are *direct* and hence not morally acceptable.

I think it is vital to stress the fact that in this response the Church is not meddling in medicine. The Congregation is saying, in effect, that the decisions to perform the hysterectomy of question two or the uterine isolation of question three are not, properly speaking, medical decisions at all. True, they can certainly *appear* to be medical and they can be carried out successfully by medical prowess, to be sure, but in reality they are *moral* in nature. This is how the Congregation phrases it:

> Therefore, the described procedures do not have a properly therapeutic character but are aimed in themselves at rendering sterile future sexual acts freely chosen. The end of avoiding risks to the mother, deriving from a possible pregnancy, is thus pursued by means of a direct sterilization, in itself always morally illicit, while other ways which are morally licit, remain open to free choice.

It is important to remember that Fr. O'Donnell made it abundantly clear that his thesis regarding the solid probability of uterine isolation revolved around one central feature, namely, that the procedure is *indirect* sterilization. O'Donnell has over and again said that he himself regarded the sole moral defense of the procedure of uterine isolation to be, as the Jesuit moralist himself puts it, "the solid probability of the moral opinion that it is not a directly contraceptive sterilization."[16] The response of the Congregation has answered *that* precise question: in the absence of an actual pathology, the sterilization must be regarded as *direct.* With this determination, the "sole moral defense of the procedure," as Fr. O'Donnell, the father of the uterine isolation issue, viewed the matter, has vanished.

A summary of some of the major points that the Congregation is making may be helpful:

1. The "weak uterus" is not a disease.[17]

2. Pregnancy is not a disease.

3 "Uterine isolation" treats no disease.

4. "Uterine isolation" is not a medical intervention.

5. "Uterine isolation" is a direct sterilization.

6. "Uterine isolation" is morally contraindicated because direct sterilization is morally contraindicated.

Pastoral Dimensions

"You can't do one thing only." In discussing the topic of uterine isolation we find ourselves touching upon crucial elements of Catholic doctrine regarding marriage and human sexuality. Far from being a minor issue, the discussion of the issues surrounding our topic has helped us to clarify what is at stake in medicine and morality.

Father Albert Moraczewski once asked in the pages of *Ethics & Medics* the question, "Whose Turf Is It Anyway?"[18] In a sense the Congregation has given the answer: cases two and three may masquerade as medicine but they are in reality moral issues.

One of the breakout sessions at our current workshop deals with the topic of Women and Health Care. In taking the position it does vis-à-vis the question of uterine isolation, is the Church playing fast and loose with the health of women? If I may employ the language of the radical feminists for a moment: Are women being sacrificed upon the altar of a masochistic male morality? If I may attempt an ever so brief answer: far from denigrating the moral agency of women, the Congregation is enhancing it with the 1993 Responses.

Case One is a medical emergency, cases two and three are moral issues. The way these issues are to be resolved is more by way of resolute human moral action than by means of surgical procedures. The courage it takes to assume the risks of a pregnancy—any pregnancy, to be sure, but especially so in cases that may not be ideal—and the courage it takes to bring a child into the world have always been accepted most graciously by our mothers and sisters who have been fashioned no less than us in the image and likeness of God.

Medical science is there to assist with its wonders, either to bring difficult pregnancies to term or else to make women aware that it can help them avoid the dangers and the risks associated with such pregnancies. Church teaching on the matter urges us to handle medical issues as medical issues, moral decisions as moral decisions. Women are free and responsible moral agents. The wonders of modern medicine can, as Dr. Goodwin intimates, "medicalize" moral decisions. While we see most clearly in the abortion debate the possibility of the medical profession providing *surgical* solutions to *social* problems, the same is true in the problematic we are discussing today, namely, uterine isolation. Medical science has all the tools available to help women through very difficult pregnancies; the same medicine can also obviate such pregnancies by means of direct contraceptive sterilization, the kind that may be provided by means of tubal ligation, a.k.a. uterine isolation.

How do free and responsible moral agents act when faced with such possibilities? Far from demeaning women's moral agency, the Church in this 659-word response places it at a very high level indeed. In a sense, women and men are both confronted by the technological imperative: the fact that we have the technology to do something—does this *ipso facto* mean that the moral question is thereby resolved? The Congregation's terse statement does not think so. Neither does the recently approved edition of the *Ethical and Religious Directives.*[19]

Health Care Professionals

The task confronting bishops and others interested in quality Catholic health care is at one and the same time a challenging, delicate, and didactic one. Health care professionals can provide, as it were, medical certitude but in the cases of hysterectomy and uterine isolation such as outlined in cases two and three the most we can have is moral rather than medical certitude. Indeed, in line with the theme of this year's Workshop, it may well turn out to be the case that the whole question boils down to the issue of freedom. The marvels of modern medicine can make us forget what the Responses urge us to consider.

Therefore, the described procedures do not have a properly therapeutic character but are aimed in themselves at rendering sterile future sexual acts freely chosen. Since it was Fr. O'Donnell who kept the discussion of uterine isolation alive, we might expect that his recent statement in the *Linacre Quarterly* that uterine isolation is unacceptable in Catholic teaching will bring an end to the fifty-year old discussion. Before we leave it, I would like to build upon his efforts in the conclusion to this workshop session.

Married Couples:
The View of Frs. Ford and Kelly
Perpetual Abstinence *or* Dangerous Pregnancy

As the discussion of uterine isolation began to take shape in the 1940s and 1950s, authors such as Frs. Ford and Kelly saw the issue as one either of perpetual abstinence or of a dangerous pregnancy.[20] Why not uterine isolation if the alternative is the foregoing of the unitive aspect of a couple's sexuality? In this regard, we are impressed with their pastoral solicitude.

What has Changed: The Management of Pregnancies
The Scientific Basis for Natural Family Planning

No longer is the alternative what Frs. Ford and Kelly thought it was: danger or abstinence. Today we can add a third element: periodic continence with a scientific basis such as we find in the modern versions of Natural Family Planning. The certitude this method grants is, truth to tell, precisely what we have come to expect from the uterine isolation problematic: moral certitude, no more, no less.

On a practical level, may I recommend that one excellent way for the uterine isolation issue to have served as a teaching moment for the Church is to see to it that the teaching of Natural Family Planning be established as a Church-wide policy for all couples as part of their marriage preparations.[21] This teaching of Natural Family Planning must include both its moral theory as well its technical aspects. Because of its dual component, the need for cooperation by the priests and the laity is readily apparent. The appreciation of both for the work of the other may well grow as a result of this collaboration.

NFP and CCL: Reworking Two Acronyms

Time was, Natural Family Planning in the eyes of some meant *Not For Progressives*. Thanks to the labors of the Billings and the Hilgers as well as the many others devoted to this work, we have grown beyond such a narrow view. Natural Family Planning is better understood to suggest "*Now and For Posterity.*"

The acronym CCL stands for the Couple-to-Couple League. May I commandeer the acronym so that it can also stand for the "Couples to Clergy League" as well? Any meaningful initiative on the values of Natural Family Planning will probably come from the laity to the clergy rather than the other way around.

Lay people will have to tell their priests and bishops that methods of artificial birth control are a dead-end. They will have to show in their lives the truth that Natural Family Planning does work. The Church has known this in theory all along. But a generation of priests has had it drummed into them that Natural Family Planning is nothing else but a new name for "rhythm" and that it does not work effectively.[22] These priests have read in their daily newspapers and heard on the TV newscasts and talk shows that only the Pill and the condom and the IUD and the diaphragm and the tubal ligations and the vasectomies and the abortions are what "the people in the pews" are living. If Catholics want to hear sermons from the pulpit once again on moral subjects that matter to couples who want to live their faith, it is up to the couples to tell the priests that Natural Family Planning works and that the devices of the sexual revolution are all dead-ends.

Several years ago at Providence Hospital in the Diocese of Springfield (MA), I took a course in Natural Family Planning, unaccompanied save for my good intentions. I attended along with approximately fifteen couples, affectionately dubbed the "granola crowd." Such efforts in dioceses around the country must continue, to be sure, but the ability to add to the Natural Family Planning lectures the theological roots of *Humanae Vitae* no. 16 and *Familiaris Consortio* no. 33 must be stressed. Without this theological component, Natural Family Planning can come across as part of the contraceptive mentality rather than as a way in which spouses can honor God with their bodies as they "fight for the work of God."

More than a decade ago, at the 1984 Dallas Workshop, Bishop McHugh and Mr. Gérard Brunelle gave an excellent presentation on NFP. Last year Australian Doctors John and Evelyn Billings did likewise. In between this topic has been dealt with over and again at Workshops and in the publications of the Pope John Center. Those who continue to speak on the topic must feel a bit like Rodney Dangerfield: "No respect, no respect at all." And yet, if "repetitio est mater studiorum," it is a message that must continue.

While the reasons for its Rodney Dangerfield status would make for an interesting discussion, I would much prefer to regard Natural Family Planning as the "Joan Rivers" of responsible parenthood: at its heart, it asks the question: "CAN WE TALK?" It asks it of spouses, it also asks it of couples and clergy. Artificial methods of birth control: the pill, the IUD, the diaphragm, the condom, sterilization of either male or female or perhaps of both, are monologues, entered into by ONE. Natural Family Planning demands dialogue as couples strive to love each other in the way God created them. Husbands and wives, priests and people, the entire community of faith: as we prepare to live our faith in the 21st century, "CAN WE TALK?"

While the fifty-year debate over uterine isolation is over, the issues it raised has helped us clarify some very important components of the Christian walk of faith. Let its very name be its epitaph: Uterine isolation? In morals as in medicine the same truth holds: You can't do one thing only.

Notes

1. This is the estimate of the situation according to Rev. Edward J. Bayer, S.T.D., "Isolating the Threatening Womb," *Ethics & Medics*, vol. 10, no. 2 (1985): 3-4.

2. Fr. John Ford, S.J. wrote of the possibility of a tubal ligation in the case of a weak uterus in 1942. See his "Current Theology: Notes on Moral Theology, 1942," *Theological Studies* 3 (1942): esp. 590-593. A Vatican statement of 1940 to the effect that direct sterilization is unacceptable because it is against the natural law would seem to be the trigger for action on uterine isolation. Jesuit moralist Fr. Gerald Kelly on several occasions brought up the 1940 statement.

3. When I say that uterine isolation is a "minor point," in no way, of course, do I intend to downplay the medical importance of the situations in which patients find themselves. Statistically, however, the number of instances where uterine isolation was envisioned as applicable by Fr. O'Donnell was always very limited.

4. See Thomas J. O'Donnell, S.J., "'Uterine Isolation' Unacceptable in Catholic Teaching," *Linacre Quarterly*, 61 (Aug., 1994): 58-61.

5. O'Connell may be overly harsh on himself, speaking as he does of "renouncing his errors." It seems to me that Fr. O'Donnell had never advanced his thesis that uterine isolation is a solidly probable opinion in a way that was anything but thoroughly faithful to the Church.

6. The article to which Fr. O'Donnell refers is that of Sister Renée Mirkes, M.A., "Uterine Isolation: A Euphemism?" *Ethics & Medics*, vol. 18, no. 1 (1993): 1-3.

7. In preparing for this presentation, I mentioned the expression "uterine isolation" to three doctors: a pathologist, a urologist, and an ob/gyn. Only the last mentioned *had* heard of the term but not, as he put it, for about twenty years. The expression is found neither in medical dictionaries nor in on-line computer medical services. While "uterine isolation" may draw a blank, "tubal ligation" was known by all three. This point is not lost in the Vatican Responses as we see in the very way the second question was posed, namely, "Is it licit to substitute tubal ligation, also called uterine isolation?"

8. Some will no doubt remember the workshop presentation, "'Medicalizing' Moral Decisions in Reproductive Medicine," delivered by Dr. Thomas Murphy Goodwin at the 1994 Bishops' Workshop. The text is found in Russell E. Smith, ed. *Faith and Challenges to the Family* (Braintree, MA: Pope John Center, 1994), 79-99.

9. On this, in addition to the aforementioned work of Dr. Goodwin, consult Thomas Hilgers, M.D., "Family Planning Issues: NFP, Norplant, Uterine Isolation,"

in *The Interaction of Catholic Bioethics and Secular Society* (Pope John Center: Braintree, MA, 1992), 213-230.

10. Goodwin, "'Medicalizing' Moral Decisions," 93.

11. If proof were needed for our oft-repeated contention that "You can't do one thing only," it may be found in the route one would have to take in coming to an understanding of some of the medical (and at times not-so-medical) aspects of the issues surrounding this problematic, involving as they do not only sterilization and tubal ligation but also uterine rupture, hysterectomy, and the question of how the medical profession has managed women's health care concerns in general. I have found the following helpful: Norman F. Miller, "Hysterectomy: Therapeutic Necessity or Surgical Racket?" *American Journal of Obstetrics and Gynecology*, 51 (1946): 804-810; Waverly R. Payne, M.D., "Hysterectomy--A Problem in Public Relations," *American Journal of Obstetrics and Gynecology*, 72 (1956): 1165-1170; John Cattanach, "Oestrogen Deficiency after Tubal Ligation," *The Lancet* (April 13, 1985): 847-849; Richard M. Farmer, M.D., Ph.D. et alii, "Uterine Rupture During Trial of Labor After Previous Cesarean Section," *American Journal of Obstetrics and Gynecology*, 165 (1991): 996-1001; Anna S. Leung, M.D., Richard M. Farmer, M.D., et alii, "Risk Factors Associated With Uterine Rupture During Trial of Labor After Cesarean Delivery: A Case-Control Study," *American Journal of Obstetrics and Gynecology*, 168 (1993): 1358-1362; M.A. Bey, et al., "Comparison of Morbidity in Cesarean Section Hysterectomy versus Cesarean Section Tubal Ligation," *Surgery, Gynecology and Obstetrics* 177 (1993): 357-360; and M. Langer et al., "Psychological Sequelae of Surgical Reversal or of IVF after Tubal Ligation," *International Journal of Fertility and Menopausal Studies* 38 (1993): 44-49. The topic of the successful management of difficult pregnancies has hit the mass-market as well. See for example Diana Hales and Timothy Johnson, M.D., *Intensive Caring: New Hope for High-Risk Pregnancy* (New York: Crown Publishers, 1990).

12. Fathers Gerald Kelly and Francis Connell were discussing the meaning of "pathology" almost from the outset of the current debate. See for example how Father Kelly saw the issue in his "Notes on Moral Theology, 1950," *Theological Studies*, 12 (1951): 68-73. On the other side, we have Francis J. Connell, C.Ss.R., "Answers to Questions: A Surgical Problem," *American Ecclesiastical Review*, 121 (1949): 507, and "Answers to Questions: Moral Problems in Surgery," *American Ecclesiastical Review*, 123 (1950): 220-1.

13. It is perhaps worth noting that the word "present" occurs three times in the Vatican statement. Some pertinent comments are made on the temporal dimensions of the Vatican statement by Peter Cataldo of the staff of the Pope John Center in his article, "Uterine Isolation: What the Vatican Says and Does Not Say," *Ethics & Medics*, vol. 19, no. 12 (1994): pp. 3-4.

14. See Macdonald Critchley, Editor-in-Chief, *Butterworths Medical Dictionary* [2nd ed.], (Butterworths: London and Boston, 1978), s.v. "Pathology," p. 1260. A helpful history of pathology is found in the first chapter, "The History and Scope of Pathology," pp. 1-20, to Sir Edwin Florey, ed. *General Pathology* [3rd ed.] (W.B. Saunder Company: Philadelphia and London, 1962); Florey himself wrote the chapter.

15. For more on this, see Cataldo's article.

16. Thomas J. O'Donnell, S.J., *Medicine and Christian Morality*, 2nd ed. revised and updated (Staten Island: Alba House, 1991), 144.

17. As we have seen, for 30 years the expression has not occurred in the medical literature. Even if we were to concede for the sake of argument the existence of a "damaged" or "weak" uterus, it seems too great a stretch to term this *condition* a *disease.* The handling of pregnancies in such cases—and in cases far more severe—is medically possible.

18. See Albert S. Moraczewski, "Whose Turf Is It, Anyway?" *Ethics & Medics*, vol. 11, no. 11 (1986): 3-4.

19. It seems to me that the "Introduction" to Part Four of the 1994 *Ethical and Religious Directives* makes excellent sense on this precise point.

20. See John C. Ford, S.J. and Gerald Kelly, S.J., *Contemporary Moral Theology. Vol. II: Marriage Questions* (Westminster, MD: Newman Press, 1963). Making the same general observation is John R. Connery, S.J., "Notes on Moral Theology," *Theological Studies*, 16 (1955): 574-577.

21. Interestingly enough, Father O'Donnell devotes a section to the topic of NFP in his 1991 *Medicine and Christian Morality*. See pp. 219-223.

22. Note how one author speaks of NFP: "Discovering whether natural family planning 'works' means running an irresponsible risk." The words belong to Richard A. McCormick, S.J., *The Critical Calling: Reflections on Moral Dilemmas Since Vatican II* (Washington, D.C.: Georgetown University Press, 1989), 280.

Chapter 5

HEALTH CARE REFORM LEGISLATION: DISAPPOINTMENTS, CURRENT PROSPECTS, AND URGENT ISSUES

Richard M. Doerflinger, M. A. Div.

My overall message about health care reform legislation is not very optimistic: Such legislation failed in the U.S. Congress last year not because the need for it diminished, but because fear and distrust of comprehensive reform became more powerful than fear of the underlying problem. The need continues and in some ways seems likely to grow—but some solutions now coming forward only tinker around the edges of the problem, while other solutions are frightening indeed.

The need for reform is clear. Over 37 million Americans (over 41 million according to one recent study) lack health insurance[1]—including a growing number of people with incomes above the poverty line, who made up 28% of the uninsured in 1993. Increasingly the costs of providing care to these people are shifted onto those who have insurance. And the cost of health care is staggering. Despite a slowdown in the rate of increase in health care prices, they are still rising about 5% a year—increasing twice as fast as general price inflation. Between 1980 and 1992, federal spending on Medicaid and Medicare increased nearly fourfold, bringing their share of federal expenditures up to 14% of the total; similar trends can be seen in state governments' spending. Simply put, our health care system serves too few, costs too much and delivers care in far too haphazard a manner.[2]

The Catholic bishops' conference of the United States has been calling for a system of guaranteed health insurance in our country since its first major statement on social justice in 1919.[3] But in 1992, it seemed the political will to attempt nationwide reform had materialized in the White House and Congress.

Many Catholics, including leaders of the Catholic Health Association, had a preference for a "single-payer" system in which the government becomes the sole vendor of health insurance. Such a bill was introduced in Congress, garnering support from some liberal Democrats. But President Clinton chose to pursue an approach in greater continuity with current practice, in which most health insurance (57% in 1993) is purchased through employers. His comprehensive reform plan mandated large employers to provide a package of standard benefits to their employees, and required smaller employers to contribute to insurance "pools" from which workers could purchase coverage. The U.S. bishops' conference did not endorse any particular mechanism for reforming the health care system to ensure universal coverage, but outlined certain broad criteria by which it would judge a final plan. As we said in one letter to Congress: "In our view, the best measure of proposed health care initiatives is the extent to which they can combine universal access to quality health care with cost control, while insuring quality care for the poor and preserving human life and dignity."[4]

One serious problem in the President's plan—a problem that kept reappearing in different forms in virtually every proposal from *either* party—was the problem of abortion coverage. From our legal analysis and from past experience we knew that open-ended phrases like "reproductive health services" and "services related to pregnancy" would be interpreted in the courts as including abortion—unless they were amended to specify otherwise. Such phrases appeared in every health care reform bill that outlined a standard package of benefits for health plans. Even bills that did not specify a standard benefits package often posed a problem: Catholic hospitals, employers and employees would be required to purchase insurance or participate in provider networks that included abortion, and would have no protection for their conscientious objection to such procedures. Many sponsors of these bills did not want to face these problems—they reasoned that any explicit policy either for or against abortion would divide the Congress and lose much-needed votes for their proposals.

But in the end, it was not primarily the issue of abortion that doomed comprehensive reform. It was increasing partisan division in Congress, fueled by a growing distrust of any active government role in decisions about health care. One may speak here of a growing conservative tide among the voters; it may more accurately be described as a growing cynicism about the federal government's ability to make a positive contribution to large social problems. As the President's plan was increasingly accused of plotting a "government takeover" of health care that would infringe on citizens' ability to choose their own doctor and insurance coverage, compromise proposals and more modest bills of all kinds multiplied—but no one of them ever achieved sufficient support to move forward as the dominant proposal.

Because it began to seem that comprehensive reform would not be possible in the short term, many members of Congress decided to settle for incremental reforms, fixing specific problems in order to reduce costs or increase access to coverage: increasing "portability" of insurance from one employer to another, providing tax benefits for the purchase of private insurance, capping punitive damages in medical malpractice suits, preventing or limiting the exclusion of people with "pre-existing conditions" from the insurance market, etc. Such proposals were far less frightening to many middle-class voters who were apprehensive about massive change in the present system—but they also failed to address major elements of the problem, and were unlikely to help the poor and vulnerable people most in need of systemic reform. Nonetheless, the new, more conservative Congress is unlikely to give serious consideration to any proposal that goes beyond such relatively minor changes.

Perhaps the most frustrating debate in which the bishops' conference had to participate last year was a dispute with several pro-life groups which share our firm opposition to abortion and euthanasia. These groups were concerned about cost pressures that could lead government to "ration" health care—in particular, to deny life-preserving treatment to seriously ill or disabled people who want such treatment and need it to survive. The concern itself was valid, as will be clear in what follows. But some groups decided that virtually *any* government intervention that tried to combine universal access with price controls would inevitably produce "rationing" of this kind. Using this argument, groups like the National Right to Life Committee came out in opposition to President Clinton's health plan and several others regardless of whether they would be amended to exclude mandated abortion coverage. When combined with politically conservative groups already committed to retaining the "free market" system as much as possible, these groups persuaded many members of Congress that comprehensive reform would cause more problems than it would solve.

There are some flaws in this claim about government rationing. For one thing, it seems clear that various kinds of rationing or deliberate denial of treatment for cost reasons goes on now, not only by government but also by health insurance companies and managed care plans trying to maintain their profit margins. Patients are checked out of the hospital "quicker and sicker" so their care will not cost more than the average amount allowed under federal DRG (diagnosis-related grouping) reimbursement policies. The patients most in need of quality health care are subjected to "red-lining" because they are seen as bad risks to the insurance industry. Expensive procedures are reviewed and frequently withheld by insurance companies using various kinds of "cost-benefit" analysis. And most frequently of all, care is effectively rationed based on income level, because so many of the working poor simply cannot afford health insurance at today's inflated prices while the wealthy can pay out of their pockets for whatever care they may need. This kind of rationing can only increase and become more pervasive if the present wasteful system is not reformed.

A second flaw in the argument is the assumption that we are operating in a "zero-sum" system, where expanding care to more people must necessarily mean providing less care to each person covered. Under such an assumption, ensuring universal access to health care will exert an extra strain on total cost, so any effort to restrain cost increases will mean denying needed care to many people. But in fact, giving everyone access to the same system may actually help solve some of the problems that now drive up costs.

In the current system, people without health insurance tend to stay away from doctors until they are in urgent need—they wait until a crisis, and then turn up in our hospital emergency rooms where treatment is extremely costly. Because they cannot pay for this care, its cost is then shifted onto those who have insurance and drives up their cost. As a result, more and more people find themselves unable to afford insurance—they join the uninsured and feed this vicious cycle all over again. The cycle could be broken if everyone were ensured basic coverage, and everyone could receive regular checkups and preventive care and contribute something into a common system. And if everyone joined the same system, the more wealthy and powerful would have an incentive to make sure the benefits available to all are reasonably generous—because they, too, would be bound by the same standard. But of course, the idea of discouraging people from "buying out" of the system with their own money was one of the proposals most fiercely criticized last year as an unwarranted restraint on personal freedom.

So universal coverage may not aggravate the cost crisis and the threat of rationing as much as some people think. The waste and inefficiency, the cost shifting, and the profiteering that go on in the present fragmented system drive up costs in their own way, without improving the availability or quality of care.

Nonetheless, Congress's attention has now shifted from health care reform to welfare reform, and perhaps to immigration—both of which are seen as related problems that help to aggravate the health care crisis. These debates may yet have some direct impact on health care in this Congress—for example, as part of the welfare reform debate, Senator Nancy Kassebaum has proposed that the federal government completely take over the Medicaid system for providing health care to the poor, and hand the welfare system over to the states. But most likely we will see this Congress do little on health care except the kind of incremental reforms mentioned earlier: tort reform and limited "market reforms" that may make it easier for some people to purchase or retain private health insurance.

This means that the states are now the focus of attention for this debate, and in fact several states have already attempted significant reforms, with mixed success. For example, some positive results can be seen in Hawaii, where efforts to achieve universal coverage have *reduced* costs instead of raising them. Hawaii now covers 98% of its citizens, and the percentage of its GNP spent on health care is less than 9% (compared with 13% for the nation).[5]

A complete account of this and other efforts is not possible here. However, one experiment by a state deserves special attention, because it is among the most ambitious and has also become the most frightening.

For several years the state of Oregon has been trying to implement a plan to ration all health care for the poor through its Medicaid program. The plan was designed to expand the number of low-income people, especially mothers and children, covered by Medicaid; the funds for this expansion would be obtained by denying payment for various treatments seen as not being cost-effective. The state created a priority list of over 600 treatments, ranked according to their estimated cost-effectiveness; in any given year, the state legislature would decide how much money is available for Medicaid, and the cutoff point would be set accordingly, so that treatments falling below the cutoff line will not be available to the poor. The state also planned to set up an "employer mandate" program requiring employers to provide insurance to their workers.

There are several serious problems with the Oregon plan. First of all, it fails the test of subjecting all citizens to the same limits—care will be rationed *only* for the poor. Some state officials who support the plan have said they would be proud to have their families covered by it—but none of them has hurried to sign up. Secondly, within the poor population it sets different populations against each other—most often, poor women and children against the poor elderly, handicapped and terminally ill for whom treatment is seen as less cost-effective. Third, the formula used to create the priority list goes beyond effectiveness in curing disease or saving life, to incorporate judgments about the "quality" of the life saved. To be sure, any health care system should concern itself with enhancing people's quality of life as much as possible. But if such judgments are used to classify some kinds of lives as not worth living, a health care reform program could be used as a tool for massive discrimination against frail and disabled people. In this regard it is noteworthy that vulnerable patients generally were not involved in creating the priority list—the "value" of a life with a disability was estimated by able-bodied citizens, not by the disabled themselves.[6]

Oregon's original proposal to restructure its Medicaid program in this way was rejected by the Bush Administration, on the grounds that it would violate the Americans with Disabilities Act forbidding state-sponsored discrimination against disabled citizens.[7] After modifying the most overtly discriminatory features of its formula, Oregon resubmitted its proposal to the new Clinton Administration and received permission to proceed. But the new plan is not doing very well: The state budget for Medicaid is in more trouble than originally projected, meaning that well over 100 of the listed 600 treatments may have to be denied to the indigent; the plan to ensure coverage for all workers has been delayed by economic and political problems.[8]

But what makes this plan the most ominous effort at reform in the country is the new element added on November 8 of last year, when the citizens of Oregon voted to legalize physician-assisted suicide for the terminally ill. The new law has not yet been allowed to go into effect because federal courts are considering the charges made in a lawsuit against it—including the charge that this law, too, violates the Americans with Disabilities Act. But this new combination of policies—rationing health care for the disabled and terminally ill, and authorizing assisted suicide for some of these same patients—deserves special attention, because it presents an extreme case of what may happen when health care policy is guided by fear of rising costs and unrestrained by any sound moral sense.

Under such a policy, indigent patients in various stages of cancer, AIDS, Alzheimer's or Lou Gehrig's disease could find themselves unable to qualify for any life-prolonging treatment—but completely eligible for free or low-cost lethal overdoses of drugs. The latter option would, of course, be promoted as a benefit to the patient and as just another "free choice" for the individual—but in effect it may be the poor patient's *only* choice, because other avenues have been closed off as too expensive.

In fact, almost immediately after the November vote to legalize the prescribing of lethal drugs for dying patients, the state's health commissioner announced that these suicide doses probably *will* be covered under Medicaid. Most likely, he said, they will be covered under the category of "comfort care," which ranks very high on the priority list.[9]

In one sense it is hard to deny that suicide pills are cost-effective—they are not expensive, and they are very effective at ensuring that the state will never have to pay for any further treatment for this individual. But we are in serious trouble if this is becoming the standard by which health care is judged. As ethicist Charles Dougherty has written:

> Nearly all observers agree that cost pressures will force future adoption of practice protocols based on patient condition, likely outcome, and cost of alternative treatments. If legal and widely acceptable euthanasia is added to this economic pressure, it is hard to imagine a future without practice protocols, a package of basic benefits, reimbursement restrictions, or cost-sharing arrangements that provide de facto incentives for the active killing of terminally ill patients. If this future should come to pass, the freedom to choose that many proponents of legalization champion will set the stage for not-so-subtle financial coercions that will determine how many of us die, especially the poor and uninsured or underinsured.[10]

In general, where health care reform is debated among policymakers, cost control rather than universal coverage has become the top priority. Much attention is being devoted to the high cost of treatment for the terminally ill—even President Clinton announced that his health plan would help control costs by encouraging patients to sign "living wills" that refuse aggressive treatment during the dying process. The issue has attracted a certain amount of misinformation and even demagoguery, as when then-Surgeon General Joycelyn Elders made the ridiculous statement that "ninety percent of all health care dollars are spent on the last 30 days of life."[11] One recent study, after careful analysis, concludes as follows: "The amount that might be saved by reducing the use of aggressive life-sustaining interventions for dying patients is at most 3.3 percent of total national health care expenditures. ...[T]his amount represents a fraction of the increase due to inflation in health care costs and less than the $50 billion to $90 billion needed to cover the uninsured population." In short, "we must stop deluding ourselves that advance directives and less aggressive care at the end of life will solve the financial problems of our health care system."[12]

As people frustrated over the cost crisis are tempted to target the old, the dying and the disabled for denial of care, one important role the Church can play is to point out that these vulnerable groups cannot and should not be treated as scapegoats for a problem that pervades our entire health care system. But the Church can and should do more. We should bring to bear our best policy thinking and the best of our moral tradition to enlighten the debate over health care rationing, which now often seems divided between those who deny the existence of the cost problem and those who would solve it with a battle-ax. The American people themselves are certainly divided and confused on the issue. In a recent poll of Minnesota citizens, for example, 63% agreed with this statement: "There are so many new, expensive treatments, surgical procedures, transplants, and medical devices that it is impossible for any insurance plan to pay for all of them." But in the same poll 85% agreed with the statement: "Everybody should have the right to get the best possible health care, as good as the treatment a millionaire gets."[13]

Our tradition does not insist on using every treatment that is technically possible, regardless of a patient's condition. We distinguish between ordinary and extraordinary (or as some prefer to say, between proportionate and disproportionate) means. We teach the calm and prayerful acceptance of death in cases where death is inevitable, and we have the love and understanding needed to know how to care for people we cannot cure. We also have a long tradition on social and economic justice, insisting that every social policy respect the demands of commutative and distributive justice: every human person should receive what is due to him or her, and social resources should be distributed fairly with special concern for the weak and powerless.

But how to bring together these two worlds—to combine, if you will, the microcosm of medical ethics and the macrocosm of economic justice?

In attempting to do so we cannot merely impose one model on the other in a simple-minded fashion. We cannot demand a "right to health care" that would be an unlimited claim by every person to every kind of treatment he or she may desire. Nor can we easily impose the model of ordinary and extraordinary means on our social system. For to call a treatment "extraordinary" has always meant that a patient is not morally bound to accept the treatment but *may* choose to accept it. And the central factor in determining whether a treatment is "ordinary means" is to assess the benefits and burdens *for that particular patient,* not some easily quantified factor that could be turned into an objective list of ordinary and extraordinary treatments. The question facing us now is: Under what circumstances can we deny a treatment even to a person who wants it and says he needs it? And how can our teaching on the equal dignity of every human life be made real and concrete in a debate which increasingly revolves around the question of which lives are not worth caring for or spending money on at all?[14]

Answers to these questions are far beyond the scope of this talk or the ability of this speaker. They are questions that deserve the attention of the best Catholic minds, as we confront a deeply flawed health care system—a system in danger of being reworked in accord with even more deeply flawed attitudes toward the dignity of life.

Notes

1. See "Over 41 million now uninsured," *American Medical News* (Feb. 13, 1995): p. 6 (summarizing a study by the Employee Benefit Research Institute).

2. For this analysis I am indebted to Patricia King, M.P.H., J.D., policy advisor at the U.S. Catholic Conference's Office of Domestic Social Development.

3. Administrative Committee of the National Catholic War Council, "Program of Social Reconstruction" (Feb. 12, 1919), para. 25; see Nolan (ed.), *Pastoral Letters of the United States Catholic Bishops* (U.S. Catholic Conference, 1984), Vol. I, 265.

4. Bishop James Malone (Chairman, Domestic Policy Committee, U.S. Catholic Conference), "Letter to Congress on National Health Care Reform," April 14, 1992, p. 4.

5. A. Newman and B. Jancin, "Hawaii Health Plan Seen as Model for National Reform," *Ob.Gyn. News* (Jan. 15, 1993): 31.

6. Bishop James Malone (Chairman, Domestic Policy Committee, U.S. Catholic Conference), "Letter to HHS Secretary Louis W. Sullivan," August 6, 1991; Press Release, "Oregon Catholic Conference Opposes State of Oregon Request for Medicaid Waiver," August 9, 1991.

7. See Michael J. Astrue, J.D., "Pseudoscience and the Law: The Case of the Oregon Medicaid Rationing Experiment," *Issues in Law & Medicine*, Vol. 9, No. 4 (Spring 1994): 375-86.

8. See "Oregon cuts not enough? More trims may be needed," *American Medical News* (March 13, 1995): 8.

9. Associated Press report of Nov. 11, 1994, quoting Dr. Paul Kirk, chairman of the Oregon Health Services Commission.

10. Charles J. Dougherty, Ph.D., "The Common Good, Terminal Illness, and Euthanasia," *Issues in Law & Medicine*, Vol. 9, No. 2 (Fall 1993): 151-166 at p. 160.

11. Quoted by Associated Press, May 17, 1994.

12. E. J. Emanuel and L. L. Emanuel, "The Economics of Dying: The Illusion of Cost Savings at the End of Life," *New England Journal of Medicine*, Vol. 330, No. 8 (Feb. 24, 1994): 540-44 at p. 543. Also see S. Rich, "Study: Denying Care to Terminally Ill is Futile," *The Washington Post*, Nov. 1, 1994, p. A7.

13. Steve Miles, M.D., "Health Care Resource Allocation," *Newsletter: The Center for Biomedical Ethics: U. of Minnesota* (Winter 1995): 1.

14. For one responsible, though not completely satisfying, attempt to answer this question see Stephen G. Post, "Health Care Rationing?" *America* (Dec. 5, 1992): 453-5.

Chapter 6

CANONICAL CONCERNS IN CATHOLIC HEALTH CARE

Nick P. Cafardi, Esq.

In the nineteenth century, great waves of Catholic immigrants came to American shores, driven by crop failures in Ireland, industrial expansion in northern and central Europe, and the fall of the kingdom of the Two Sicilies in Italy. These immigrants came to work the steel mills, coal mines, railroads, and factories of the New World. They were not educated people and they were very poor. They made their bread by "the sweat of their face." They found themselves in a strange land, often unable to speak the language. In their illness, they could turn to neither government nor employer who cared little for them. They could only turn to their families and their Church.

So often the Church was present in those heroic religious women and men and in the immigrant priests who accompanied the waves of newcomers to American shores. Spontaneously, reacting to human need out of the age-old Catholic tradition of the corporal and spiritual works of mercy, these religious women and men and diocesan clergy founded and staffed institutions to care for the sick and infirm immigrant. These heroic founders knew that the Church must care for these persons, not so much because no one else would, although that was the case, but because as the visible presence of Christ on this earth, they had to.

Thus, in the midst of the industrial squalor of nineteenth century America, the great Catholic institutions of health care were born. There is no doubt that, at their inception, they were the activity of the religious or diocesan groups to which their founders belonged. These founders gave little thought to legal structure. Indeed, given the legal immunity of charities then in effect, there was little need to. They saw human need and they met it, as religious members of religious institutes and as clergy of the new American dioceses.

It is about these great Catholic organizations of health care that I want to talk to you about today from a canonical perspective. Over the decades, the charities that these men and women founded have been incorporated and have grown; indeed, in many instances they have become multi-corporate entities delivering health care in the most modern of settings. In considering them, from a canonical perspective as they exist today, we cannot forget the roots of these institutions, namely, that these activities were carried on by women and men acting on behalf of the juridic persons of which they were members and priests, that these activities were considered a part of the sponsoring juridic person. They were so historically and they are so today.

In the practical application of this conclusion, the canonical concept of patrimony, or more appropriately stable patrimony, is the first item that we have to consider. Every juridic person needs stable patrimony. In fact, the *Code of Canon Law* says that juridic persons are not to be established unless they have the "resources necessary to achieve their ends" (c. 114, 3). That's interesting, isn't it, because we don't automatically think of juridic personality in terms of property, but there it is in canon 114—don't establish a juridic person without the basic property that it needs to fulfill its ends. And look at the qualification on the type of property, not just any kind of property, but property needed to fulfill its ends.

Just as no juridic person is to be established without essential assets, no juridic person is to be established unless it has a purpose that is "congruent with the mission of the Church" (c. 114, 1). This is the juridic person's end or finality—a purpose congruent with the mission of the Church—to which the property required of the juridic person is to be ordered. You can see the inevitable logic of the *Code* building here. No juridic person is to be established without assets essential to achieve its ends, and those ends must be a purpose that is congruent with the mission of the Church. So the essential property of a juridic person is really the property that the juridic person needs to achieve the purpose for which it was established. This is another way of describing stable patrimony, although the *Code* doesn't use that term in canon 114, but the reference is obvious. The property that a juridic person needs to achieve the ends for which it was established is the stable patrimony of the juridic person. It keeps it, it uses it for the proper purposes and it hands it on to future generations. Without this property, the juridic person could not exist, for it would not have the means necessary to achieve its ends.

Applying this notion of stable patrimony to the health care field, it logically follows that, when an end or purpose of a religious institute is the care of the infirm, then the assets that it needs to meet this end comprise the stable patrimony of the institute. In the case of diocesan hospitals, health care is not a solitary purpose of the diocese, but it can be a purpose if that choice has been made historically, in which case the assets necessary to achieve that end are a part of the diocese's stable patrimony.

I think that there is a kind of elegant logical neatness that the *Code* creates here—examine the ends of the juridic person and you can tell what its stable patrimony is. There is just one slight refinement needed to make the concept complete. The 1983 *Code* says that stable patrimony is stabilized through an act of "lawful designation." In other words, stable patrimony doesn't just happen. Some juridic act is necessary on the part of the juridic person to place property in the stable patrimony category. It should not happen by implication. Certainly there can be a formal act whereby property is stabilized—creating a foundation or a restricted fund for example. More likely than not, that will not be the case, however. What will happen most often is that a juridic person, by specifically dedicating property to one of its essential ends, will thereby make it a part of stable patrimony.

Some tracing or tracking of assets is appropriate here. Not every piece of property that a juridic person holds for its health care apostolate is a part of the juridic person's stable patrimony. For example, the juridic person itself may, at the time of acquisition, specify that this is an investment property, and despite its use in the apostolate, is not to be considered a part of stable patrimony. That is quite possible. In other cases, there may be accretions to the original stable patrimony that notions of fairness and justice keep out of the stable patrimony category; for example, federal funds that may come to a hospital, not as fees for services, but as grants for capital improvements, or even community funds, donated for the purposes of health care but in no way intended to accrue to the sponsor. Such accretions would not be a part of stable patrimony. Fees for services, to the extent they are used to acquire further assets, could generate stable patrimony. Fees for services are not grants and the hospital has the right to use such income without further claim from anyone.

I have no doubt that when a diocese or a religious institute took steps in the late nineteenth or early twentieth century to give a manageable corporate form to individual health care apostolates, the very corporate form itself became a part of the enduring patrimony of the institute. The reason for this categorization is quite simple: the corporate form was necessary to carry out the apostolate. It was an essential element. Now corporations are obviously property. Under American law, business corporations have equitable owners called stockholders; non-profit corporations do not have owners, but they do have controlling parties, either the members of the corporation, or the board, or a combination of both.

For those organizations that are canonically Catholic, and without some demonstrable reason as to why the general model does not fit them, I presume most hospitals that identify themselves as Catholic are so canonically, i.e., they have been founded by a public juridic person as a part of that person's apostolate and they remain part of the sponsoring public juridic person. Then the hospital's corporate identity and that part of the hospital's stable assets that are necessary to fulfill the function of a hospital, to carry out the end of health care, are a part of the stable patrimony of the public juridic person, and as such are subject to the Church's law on their use and alienation. Once an institution is recognized as canonically Catholic, that it is Catholic because it shares the public juridic personality of its sponsor, then its stable assets that have their source in the sponsor, or in the natural growth of the enterprise, are a part of the patrimony of the sponsor.

There will be times when some stable assets of a Catholic hospital or hospital system are not a part of patrimony—they were contributed by the state or by the local citizenry for a specific purpose—or the religious sponsor never took ownership but simply agreed to administer the facility. There may even be some times when changes were made in the hospital's corporate structure that had the legal effect of severing the ties between the founding sponsor and the hospital. Very often there was no canonical approval of these civil law developments, and as a result we probably have what could be termed an involuntary alienation. Very often these happened in the utmost good faith—recall there was a period following the publication of the McGrath thesis and before any learned response to it when canonists were telling religious sponsors that these incorporated institutions were no longer a juridic part of the Church and that the rules on alienation did not apply. And now many of these are irretrievably lost. Obviously alienated property, even improperly alienated property, is no longer a part of patrimony. But these are, we hope, the exception, not the rule.

Just as often, these hospitals, now absent of any effective canonical ties to the Church because of the improper alienation, still refer to themselves as Catholic and they certainly could be. Their property, having been unwittingly alienated, may no longer qualify as the stable patrimony of the sponsoring public juridic person, but they represent themselves as Catholic, they agree to be bound by the *Ethical and Religious Directives*, and just as importantly, the local bishop recognizes this fact and agrees that, yes, this is a Catholic institution.

Now such hospitals may not be canonically Catholic in the sense that they have no clear juridic category into which they fit—they are not their own public juridic person, they do not share the juridic personality of another juridic person, they lack the statutes and the recognition of an association, but they are Catholic, and, this is important, they are nonetheless subject to the Church's laws. You do not have to have a recognizable canonical existence or clear canonical ties to the Church in order to be Catholic in a meaningful legal sense.

The primary difference between such *de facto* Catholic hospitals and those hospitals that remain a part of the sponsoring public juridic person is that their property is not the patrimony of a public juridic person. As a result, the rules on alienation will not apply, because the proper object of alienation is the stable patrimony of a public juridic person. But other rules do apply, and these rules are primarily the *Ethical and Religious Directives.* A hospital that calls itself Catholic, without any clear canonical ties to the Church, or a hospital that perhaps once had those ties but severed them through an alienation, whether properly done or not, can only remain Catholic if it stays faithful to the *Directives.* This call belongs to the local diocesan bishop. The *Code* says that he is the one in his diocese to say what is and what is not Catholic, and it seems to me to be a very logical trade-off that for non-canonical hospitals he require fidelity to the *Directives* as the minimal price for the hospital to maintain this important designation as a Catholic hospital.

In this regard, there is an interesting canonical development occurring in Catholic health care in which bishops are being asked to recognize as private juridic persons a lay association which has as its purpose the operation of a Catholic health care facility. This situation has developed because of the simple lack of numbers of religious men and women in the health care apostolate who are interested and able to manage Catholic hospitals in the more traditional manner, namely as incorporated apostolates of their religious communities. In this void, Catholic laypersons are stepping forward and saying, "Let us do it." And they want to do it as a part of the Church, with some official status.

In such a situation, a local bishop could certainly erect this association as a private juridic person, provided certain safeguards are in place. First and foremost, the bishop has to review the statutes of the organization and ascertain that they are suitable to a private juridic person. They must have a purpose that is congruent with the mission of the Church. They must agree to act in accordance with the *Directives*. They must agree to be bound by the canons in their activities. They must accept ecclesiastical authority.

But if these safeguards are in place, then there would appear to be no reason not to encourage this development. Because they are private and not public juridic persons, their property cannot be considered Church property, as is that of a public juridic person, so notions of patrimony and alienation are never at issue. And because they are private, not public juridic persons, they do not act officially in the name of the Church the way a public juridic person does. But they are Catholic organizations, and they are bound by the law of the Church.

At the present time, our health care delivery system is under intense pressure from the government, and from private insurers, to greatly reduce costs. The drive to reduce costs can cause many difficulties for Catholic hospitals, difficulties that are not just economic. For example, there is great pressure now to combine services and to constrict assets. A community that needs only two hundred hospital beds is not well served by two hospitals that together provide it with three hundred beds. Someone is paying for the cost of those unfilled and unnecessary extra hundred beds, namely the patients in the two hundred beds that are filled.

More and more Catholic hospitals are being asked to join forces with non-Catholic hospitals in an attempt to create economies of scale that will drive down health care costs. Sometimes market forces even lead to the possibility of the Catholic hospital jointly offering services with the non-Catholic hospital or even merging with it. Joint ventures are the more easily manageable of these two endeavors. Agreeing to jointly own a movable MRI unit or to share laundry, pharmacy or computing services with other hospitals present very few canonical issues. Obviously such joint ventures should be structured legally so that the Catholic identity and the patrimony of the Catholic hospital are not placed in jeopardy.

A more serious problem for Catholic hospitals today is the merger question. You may think that mergers are a matter of choice between merging hospitals, but in today's health care delivery system, mergers do not always involve free choice. More and more we are seeing that mergers are forced upon smaller hospitals because they cannot compete in a stand-alone position. Alliances have to be formed, primarily by decree of the insurance industry, although I am sure that you will recall that a major component of the President's failed health care plan was the creation of these health care alliances as well.

I personally represented a small, stand-alone Catholic hospital. The hospital was struggling; it had few HMO contracts, and occupancy was limping along at about 30 to 35 per cent of capacity. And to make matters worse, only a handful of the religious women whose institute had founded the hospital were interested in the health care apostolate. The handwriting was on the wall. The hospital was about to close. At this time, we were approached by a group of five other hospitals, one Catholic, two Lutheran, a Baptist and a private non-denominational hospital, to merge and create a multi-hospital system. If we did not agree to the merger, they were prepared to build a competing hospital in the same suburb, so the hospital that I represented agreed to the merger. Did we have a choice? No, practically speaking we did not. And one of the toughest parties to deal with was the other Catholic hospital who had committed to the merger before talking to us.

This is the kind of thing that is happening in health care today. The negotiations for the merger were onerous. We went around and around the bush with our merger partners on a number of sensitive issues. Because of their own religious background, there was no question about abortions at any of the merged sites. That was barely discussed, but one of the hospitals was doing some fertility work that was clearly in violation of the *Directives;* a number of the others had no policy whatsoever on non-therapeutic tubal ligations and did not want to impose one. It was clear that the merged entity would be delivering health care services in violation of the *Directives.* Our persuasive powers on this issue were negligible, and I must admit that every time we cited Roman Catholic theology as to why we objected to certain issues, what we got back was Protestant theology that was just as well developed but that reached contrary conclusions.

We finally determined that there was no way that the Catholic hospital that I represented could participate in the final corporate structure that was going to come out of the merger. The issue of material cooperation in acts that would be violative of the *Directives* was simply insurmountable. Finally, my client simply asked to be bought out by the new merger, and that is what happened. Naturally, as a part of the buy-out process, we went to the Holy See and asked for and got alienation permission. The local bishop gave us his favorable *votum*. We had been in touch with him all along, so he appreciated the bind that the Sisters who sponsored the hospital were in.

This anecdote portrays some of the very real problems with mergers in today's health care climate. First of all, they are not necessarily something that all of the parties may want to do or choose to do. In some cases, the option is forced on them, either by competitors, by insurance companies, by harsh economic reality, or by a combination of these circumstances. Secondly, in attempting to put a merger together, certainly two critical questions will be what kinds of medical services the merged entity will be providing, and whether any of these services are violative of the *Directives*. If they are, this issue has to be addressed.

Some parties have devised interesting solutions to this issue, but they almost always involve some civil law mechanism in which the prohibited procedures are done in space that is not owned or operated by the merged entity. This results in situations where, for example, one tower in a building is the Catholic tower and another is the non-Catholic or public tower, and the non-therapeutic tubal ligations are performed in the non-Catholic space. And by the way, non-therapeutic tubal ligations or voluntary sterilization appears to be the most common sticking point, not abortions. Very few hospitals in the United States perform abortions; that has become pretty much a free-standing clinic issue. But it is not uncommon for hospitals to do tubal ligations. Whether these types of compromises work or not, I am not sure. These are, however, more issues of moral theology than they are of canon law, although the use of patrimony in a way that would violate the *Directives* is canonical as well.

Recently you may have heard that Cardinal Bernardin has issued a "Protocol" governing Catholic health care facilities in the Archdiocese of Chicago. This protocol cites his authority as diocesan bishop under canons 394 and 678 to coordinate the works of the apostolate within the archdiocese. The Protocols deal specifically with mergers and joint ventures between Catholic and non-Catholic health care facilities. The Cardinal states that, as a matter of policy, Catholic health care facilities are to collaborate with other Catholic health care facilities in preference to non-Catholic ones, and any collaboration with for-profit facilities or sale to a for-profit organization is ruled out.

The difficulty, of course, is that, even though Protocols such as the Cardinal's are a good idea—no Catholic hospital should have to face the situation that I told you about where a small Catholic hospital was forced into a merger because, among other things, it was never consulted by the larger Catholic hospital in the same market—they may not be long in effect. Certainly bishops have the right to make such rules or particular legislation for their individual dioceses when they are attempting to coordinate the various aspects of a multi-institutional apostolate, and stating a clear preference that Catholic hospitals prefer business and merger situations with other Catholic facilities where there is not that chance of loss of identity is an intelligent idea.

As good as the idea of such legislation may be, though, I am not certain of its practical effect for a number of reasons. The first is that the horse may have already left the barn. A lot of the smaller Catholic hospitals that were subject to the immense economic pressures that I have described have already succumbed or merged into non-Catholic multi-corporate forms. Secondly, the available canonical sanctions are such that, if the desire to merge or even the necessity to merge is there, they will not really stop the process. Thirdly, the imposition of such penalties will have to be done in a way that guarantees the due process rights of the sponsors.

I think that the steps taken by the Archbishop of Chicago do point his brother bishops in the right direction. As we have already seen, the pressures on Catholic hospitals in the present day health care climate are intense. Unless they are already a part of a multi-hospital Catholic system, they are on a daily basis being faced with demands that point or even coerce them in the direction of joint ventures and mergers with non-Catholic hospitals. Such steps could eventually lead to a loss of a local Catholic health care identity.

Bishops who, under their canonical authority to oversee the works of the apostolate in their diocese, are proactive in insisting on a united Catholic health care response to such challenges can help to prevent such losses. One possible response is legislative action as in Chicago. That certainly gets everyone's attention and underlines how serious this question is. But there are other tacks that can be taken as well.

The bishop is the chief pastor of his diocese. He has the authority under the *Code* to coordinate the apostolic works that are performed in his diocese. Note that this is not a property power. It is a pastoral power, a father looking out for his family. Certainly the provision of health care by the incorporated apostolates of public juridic persons within his diocese is the type of apostolic work that he is charged with overseeing. This perhaps is the most important message that I could convey today: Use your episcopacy to protect Catholic health care. Speak out when you see that it is endangered. Guide your people in seeking creative solutions to the problems that they face. Be proactive in determining that those Catholic health care institutions born of the needs of the nineteenth century endure into the twenty-first.

Chapter 7

THE DEVELOPMENT OF MORAL DOCTRINE: CHANGE AND THE UNCHANGING

The Reverend Benedict M. Ashley, O.P.

The *Catechism of the Catholic Church* says,[1]

The natural law is *immutable* and permanent throughout the variations of history; it subsists under the influx of ideas and customs and supports their progress. The rules that express it remain substantially valid. Even when it is rejected in its very principles, it cannot be destroyed or removed from the heart of man. It always rises again in the life of individuals and societies.

Veritatis Splendor, speaking of those who "question *the immutability of the natural law* itself, and thus the existence of 'objective norms of morality' valid for all people of the present and the future, as for those of the past,"[2] replies by quoting the same statement of *Gaudium et Spes*[3] referred to in the *Catechism*:

> The Church affirms that underlying so many changes there are some things which do not change and are *ultimately founded upon Christ* who is the same yesterday and today and forever.

But it then says,[4]

> Certainly there is a need to seek out and to discover *the most adequate formulation* for universal and permanent moral norms in the light of different cultural contexts, a formulation most capable of ceaselessly expressing their historical relevance, of making them understood and of authentically interpreting their truth. This truth of the moral law—like that of the 'deposit of faith'—unfolds down the centuries: the norms expressing that truth remain valid in their substance, but must be specified and determined '*eodem sensu eademque sententia*' in the light of historical circumstances by the Church's Magisterium, whose decision is preceded and accompanied by the work of interpretation and formulation characteristic of the reason of individual believers and of theological reflection.

Thus, we are faced with making the difficult distinction between the unchanging "substance" of the moral law and its historically changing "formulation." In this brief essay I will only attempt (1) to explain why the substance of the moral law cannot change, but its formulation by the Church must change; (2) to describe the principal factors promoting such historical developments; (3) to exemplify these developments, both positive and negative, in two areas of moral doctrine today hotly debated.

Only One Lord and One Community

The theological reasons that the moral law which all Christian must obey is one and unchanging are fourfold: First, God, "who wills everyone to be saved and to come to the knowledge of the truth" (1

Tm 2:4), has called all human beings to one and the same ultimate *goal*, a share in the life of the Holy Trinity. Since the moral law prescribes the means by which this goal can be reached and forbids actions that lead to dead ends, some of these means must be essential to its attainment.

Second, to reach that goal we must be *transformed* by the same Christian virtues of faith, hope, and above all love, which alone conform us to Jesus (I Cor 13:13), God's perfect image (2 Cor 4:4; Col 1:15; Heb 1:3), the "New Adam" (1 Cor 15: 22-23, 45-49). Since Jesus in his compassionate love is the unique model for Christians, the moral law must be essentially one.

Third, this form of Christian morality has for its *subject* human persons, and since all human persons are called to be incorporated in the Body of Christ, the Church (Col 1:24; Eph 1:23-30), all are called to form one community acting in harmony according to one moral law leading to the Kingdom of God.

Fourth, Christian moral life as a pilgrimage toward one single goal is empowered by the one Holy Spirit which Christ has sent from the Father, and which is, as St. Thomas Aquinas shows,[5] the New Law of grace in the hearts of the baptized (Ti 3:5) moving them to that end (Rom 5:5), and conforming them to Christ both in his humanity and in his divinity as a member of the Triune Community.

Moreover, since Jesus, our moral exemplar in the order of grace, though truly God, is also fully human, the moral law is one not only in its graced or divinized form but also as it is natural law.[6] All human beings throughout history are of one species and form one natural community. The great historic variety of languages and cultures is grounded in this unity of nature and presupposes it, because it is only because by nature we are intelligent and free that we can satisfy our essential human needs in such a variety of inventive ways.

This basic unity of humanity in its nature and predestination is the very reason for our human "historicity," why we and our moral obligations, essentially transcending time and place, are also necessarily subject to change and development. If there was no unity to the human community, it could not have a history in the proper sense of the term, because history is a shared memory, a tradition. A tradition is handed down from one generation to the next, and each generation has to reclaim it as its own in terms of its own experiences which although they have much in common with those of previous generations, are also new and unique.

Thus the moral law must be relearned and applied anew by every generation. For one generation simply to hand on that law in a particular formulation is insufficient unless the next generation understands and assimilates that essential law in its own terms. That assimilation and reformulation may be an enrichment or deepening or purification of insight, in which case we can speak of a *positive* development, or it may be an obscuration, distortion, or adulteration of that tradition, in which case we must acknowledge a *negative* development or regression.

Some exaggerate the historicity of morals to the point that all moral truths become relative to time, place, and culture. Others, more moderately, hold for transcendent "values," but deny that the categorical expression of these values can apply in all circumstances. *Veritatis Splendor* rejects both first position (*moral relativism*), and the second (*proportionalism*) as inconsistent with the universality of Jesus' moral teaching.[7]

We can conclude, therefore, that the unchanging "substance" of Christian morals is to be "perfect as your heavenly Father is perfect (Mt 5:48)," i.e., conformed to the image of God's Son who is the "image of God, the 'New Adam'," in whom the Creator's original design for our human nature is restored.

> All of us, gazing with unveiled face on the glory of the Lord, are being transformed into the same image from glory to glory, as from the Lord who is the Spirit. (2 Cor 3:18)

The Development and Retrogression of Moral Teaching

How then do positive and negative developments in moral teaching take place without changing its substance? Some today oppose two types of ecclesiology. One is a *vertical*, centralized model in which God's Word descends from on high to the Magisterium, the *ecclesia docens* to be transmitted and passively received by the faithful, the *ecclesia discens*. The other is a *concentric* model in which the Holy Spirit speaks directly to all the members of the Church while the central Magisterium merely promulgates their consensus. But is either model adequate to describe the Church in its historical development?

Certainly the concentric model helps to explain one aspect of doctrinal development. The Holy Spirit does indeed speak directly to all the baptized, enlightening every Christian who listens to the Word of God and strives to obey it. "But when he comes, the Spirit of truth, he will guide you to all truth" (Jn 16:13; cf. Acts 2:16-21, quoting Joel 3:1-5). Every member of the Church contributes something to the Church's ongoing effort to witness to the Gospel and hence to develop its moral, as well as its doctrinal teaching. Special contributions to this development are made by Christian mystics, theologians, ministers, politicians, the married, the persecuted, the suffering, etc.—not only Catholics but all Christians. We can learn and have learned from atheists and secularists. Truth, wherever found, is from the Holy Spirit. In this respect, therefore, development is concentric and centripetal, moving toward synthesis and consensus.

But obviously, in a fallen world the process of development is not merely positive. In its mission to our contemporary world the Church encounters a mentality shaped by the "knowledge explosion" and rapid technological progress. We may be "post-moderns," but the myth of "inevitable progress" still influences our thinking. Therefore, to say the moral law is "unchanging" means to many that it is as obsolescent as last year's computer software. When John XXIII called on Vatican II to "update" the Church, many took this to mean that the Ten Commandments were to be replaced with a high-tech morality.

Yet the miseries of a sinful world often lead the members of the Church to resist or neglect authoritative teaching, and sometimes Church authorities themselves neglect to teach or they teach one-sidedly or ineffectively. Hence, development of doctrine, especially on moral questions, can be regressive.

What guarantees, then, that these negative developments in the doctrinal understanding of the Church have not distorted the unchanging substance of the Gospel beyond recognition? Those who opt for a purely concentric model of development fail to give any realistic answer to this crucial question. Some, especially academics and the public media, put their faith in freedom of speech on the great principle "the truth is mighty, and will prevail." That saying would hold in a world where authentic dialogue and genuinely free and full discussion are common. That is not our world, in which self-serving propaganda, rather than truth, so often prevails.

God, therefore, in his mercy has provided in His Son, and in those whom the Son has chosen in his Church "to bind and to loose" in his name (Mt 16:19), the authority to pass judgment on the truth of teaching. Christian pastors have the responsibility to discern between what is positive and what is negative in the developments of thought and expression which flow from the whole Church to its center. Thus a sound ecclesiology rejects any separation between the horizontal or concentric aspect and the vertical or hierarchic aspect of doctrinal development. The Church as a whole in all its members engages in a process of life and reflection which leads to both positive developments born of the Holy Spirit and negative developments produced by the spirit of the world.

Of course this does not mean that the discernment of spirits is the responsibility of the Magisterium alone. Every Christian must seek the authentic Word of God. "Test everything, retain what is good" (1 Th 5:21). But the guidance of the whole Church on the right path is the responsibility of the pastors of the Church which they cannot responsibly leave simply to free discussion. They should seek ways to foster free and fair discussion, but in the end they must pass judgment on its results. And in some cases where discussion becomes more confusing and divisive than fruitful, they ought to call for a time of silent and mature reflection. At the first council of the Church in Jerusalem, after the issue of the observance of the Law by Gentile converts had been hotly debated, and Peter had spoken, we read that "The whole assembly fell silent, and they listened..." (Acts 15:12). Our age of clamorous protest forgets that truth requires a quiet growing time.

Resistance to magisterial teaching by the faithful cannot nullify its authority, although it should be the occasion for pastoral efforts to present that teaching more effectively.

Thus, human fallibility and sinfulness cannot corrupt the infallible transmission of the Gospel, but may cause it to be hidden "under a bushel basket," as Jesus warned (Mt 5:15).

The Unchanging Substance of
Sexual and Social Teaching

Catholic liberals often praise magisterial documents on social justice, but deplore their allegedly outdated views on sexual morality. Conservative Catholics praise and deplore the converse. Actually, the magisterium presents sexual morality as an essential factor in social justice, because the family is the basic institution of society, and recognizes that the family cannot flourish in an unjust society.

The Magisterium has always taught and now teaches positively in *Gaudium et Spes, Familiaris Consortio,* and the *Catechism* that God created man and woman for each other in order to manifest Christ's love for his people and to transmit this good life to future generations by a covenant of fruitful love. In the complementary roles that constitute the natural family society, each may assist all to attain holiness and eternal life. Negatively, it follows that all use of genital sex outside marriage and any use within marriage which contradicts the essential unitive and procreative purpose of the Creator is always morally wrong.

As regards social justice, the Magisterium has always taught and now teaches positively in the documents just mentioned and in many others that God created us social beings to aid each other to achieve a good human life on earth and enter together into the Kingdom of God. Hence social institutions, both church and state, must be so constructed and operated according to the principles of subsidiarity and participation as to serve this common good by protecting the rights and serving the material and spiritual needs of all their members. We members of church and state according to our different gifts must serve our neighbors for the common good. The common good of the state is the earthly flourishing of its members in virtue. The common good of the church is their union with God in Christ and the Holy Spirit. The goals of church and of the state differ but complement each other.

Negatively, the Church has always taught that abuse of institutional power, whether in church or state, for private aggrandizement instead of for the common good, and every violation of another's rights or neglect of their needs, is always immoral.

Positive and Negative
Developments of Doctrine on Sexuality

Some trace the development trajectory of doctrine on sexuality from a social emphasis on procreation to a personalistic emphasis on the intimate love between couples.[8] On this basis some also argue the "particularly significant values" to be realized in sexual behavior are that it be "self-liberating, other-enriching, honest, faithful, socially responsible, life-serving, joyous." They ask only that these positive values balance any negative values of behavior by the "principle of proportionate reason."[9]

The Magisterium, on the other hand, has regarded such developments as conformity to regressive tendencies in modern culture inimical to the family. Throughout history the Church's defense of the family has met resistance.[10] To the Jews, this teaching seemed too other-worldly, to the Gnostics too worldly. It was opposed by Greco-Roman paganism, by barbarian tribalism, by the dynastic concerns of medieval aristocracy, by the resurgent paganism of the Renaissance, by the pessimism of the Protestant reformers and Jansenists. Now it is now attacked by the secular humanism of our times when our urban economy has diminished the family's functions.

In the face of this resistance four positive developments especially stand out. First, the Church has made Jesus' teaching on the equality of the sexes in permanent covenantal monogamy a socially practical institution.[11] Only gradually and with difficulty did the sacramental nature of marriage emerge and receive public and juridical enforcement. A recent development has been the recognition by the marriage courts of the psychological conditions of a valid marriage contract.

Second, the Church has given institutional forms to the practice of virginity and celibacy for the sake of the kingdom, exemplified by the prophet Jeremiah (Jer 16:1-4), Jesus, Mary, and Paul. Furthermore, when conditions in a fallen world make marriage impossible for certain persons, Christians accept the cross of necessary abstinence with courage. Thus, for the Christian, the value of sexuality has been relativized, and many have freely chosen a consecrated celibate life, or celibacy for the sake of diaconal and priestly ministry.[12]

In our times economic pressure and the advance of medical knowledge have also commended the periodic practice of abstinence within marriage for the sake of responsible parenthood. We have also come to recognize that a homosexual orientation is not necessarily a reflection of vice, but often a genetic or developmental disadvantage. Hence the Church recommends and supports an honorable celibacy for such persons.

Third, the Church, reflecting on the modern trend to privatize sexuality by reducing it to a romantic relationship divorced from the family, has begun to emphasize the more personal, spiritual aspect of marriage, its unitive meaning. As *Familaris Consortio* insists, children have a right to be born in a family which is a school of love. This enriched theology of marriage, however, in no way, neither in *Gaudium et Spes*, nor in *Humanae Vitae*, nor in the remarkable instructions of John Paul II, who in the whole history of the papacy deserves the title *Doctor Matimonialis*, subordinates procreation to love, but instead shows that truly sexual love, by the very fact that it shares in God's creative love, is a fruitful love cooperating with the Creator to complete his human family.

A fourth development in the magisterial teaching on sexuality is a heightened compassion for those who struggle with sexual problems, whether abuse within marriage, divorce, or sexual deviations and addictions. Making use of modern sociology, psychology, and medicine to understand the causes of sexual misconduct, the Church seeks not simply to condemn it, but to seek its healing.

The development of the Church's teaching on social justice has had an even more complicated history. In the New Testament the norms of sexual morality are relatively clear and concrete while political principles are very general and implicit. The early Church was a persecuted Church without a recognized role in the social order, though it was powerfully influential within the domestic circle.

Some examples of negative developments in Catholic social practice are all too notorious. The early, underground Church rejected the use of force in its mission, but when it emerged from underground in the beginning of the fourth century, it entered into the "Constantinian Establishment" as a state church, and took on many of the questionable features of secular government, including the use of force to maintain imperial or national religious uniformity. It even adopted the legal procedures of Roman Law, including the use of torture to obtain confessions of heresy. It was only with Vatican II's *Declaration on Religious Freedom* that this centuries long regressive development was overcome.

There were, however, many positive developments, some as a result of the Church having assumed these political responsibilities, such as the gradual elimination of the institution of slavery which the New Testament had still tolerated. With the opening of the New World, in the sixteenth and seventeenth centuries, such Spanish theologians as Francis Vitoria and Bartolomé de las Casas initiated a remarkable advance in international law and the conception of universal human rights supported by the Magisterium. In the eighteenth century the Church was confronted with the counter-Christian Enlightenment and its doctrine of freedom and human rights grounded not in God's wisdom and will but in man-made constitutions and courts of law. This secularism then took the form of free-market Liberalism on the one hand, and various kinds of Socialism on the other.

On the part of a beleaguered Church, there was considerable retrogressive resistance to the secular new emphasis on human rights and a clinging to the older state patronage of the church. Beginning with Leo XIII, however, the Church has gradually elaborated a social doctrine which founds human rights in the dignity of the person created in God's image. In this development theologians and lay leaders have played a considerable part. Certainly, the theologies of liberation, in particular, have made the Church more keenly aware of the close connection of evangelization and social justice. The Magisterium, for its part, has carried out their responsibility of discernment with great prudence, steering the Bark of Peter between extremes, between the Scylla and Charibdys of *laissez-faire* and socialism, individualism and totalitarianism, technocracy and egalitarianism, radical feminism and sexism.

Twentieth century culture, which has been dominated by the United States, is essentially based, both in its conservative as well as its liberal versions, on the autonomy of individuals, each of whom seeks the maximum freedom to determine her or his manner of life. Even modern totalitarian systems have been at heart the product of this individualistic or anarchistic will-to-power. Democratic government is also intended to protect this autonomy. Political conservatives believe that this is best achieved by reducing the functions of government to defending the nation and to preventing one individual from encroaching on the privacy of another. Political liberals believe that since libertarian policies in fact deprive a considerable part of the population of their autonomy, it requires to be protected by government; while conservatives argue that such government intervention prevents these marginals from becoming autonomous members of the society. Catholic social doctrine, which is grounded not in individualism but in the inseparable love of God and neighbor, is developing in the face of this culture and often suffers from its influence either in conservative or liberal form. It rejects the notion that true freedom means the autonomy of the individual. A free society is possible only if all members accept their solidarity and that means that they accept the laws of the Creator and those of society which aim at the common good. Our freedom is one of positive responsibility and service to others. Against liberals the Church maintains the principle of subsidiarity which distributes social authority throughout the society. Against conservatives the Church rejects the notion that social justice is to be left to the working of the free market. Against both, the Church maintains the responsibility of all for each. Such broad principles, however, require to be incarnated with the same clarity as the Church's teaching on sexuality and the family. We need to place all our resources concentrically to the development of concrete social policies. This is especially the task of the laity, but under the discriminating oversight of the Church.

John Paul II in his *Tertio Millenio Adveniente* has opened up a wide vista on the great opportunities for the Church in the coming millennium as we move toward a one-world future, where cultural pluralism and global unity, along with new forms of ecological technology and biological control, become our challenge situation, along with threats of new forms of violence and contempt for human life.

Conclusion

The general conclusion which can be drawn from this brief sketch of the development of the Church's moral teaching in two difficult areas is as follows:

(1) Positive development results from a constant *resourcement*, a return to the sources to achieve a deeper understanding of the Word of God manifested fully in Jesus Christ and known to us through Scripture and Tradition. We must recover the full riches of God's Word, freed from historical one-sidedness or distortion.

(2) Negative development results from our temptation to succumb to the limited perspectives of our time and culture, whether these are "conservative," resistant to changing what is changeable, or "liberal," anxious to change even the tried-and-true. We must, indeed, mediate the Gospel to our times, but to do so we must avoid the temptation to reduce the Gospel to only what the "itching ears" (2 Tm 4:3)[13] of our contemporaries, conservative or liberal, like to hear.

Notes

1. *Catechism*, n. 1958.
2. *Veritatis Splendor*, n. 53.
3. *Gaudium et Spes*, n. 10.
4. *Veritatis Splendor*, n. 53.
5. S. Th., I-II, q. 106.
6. Some recent writers have attempted to restrict the Church's authority to revealed doctrine, thus excluding matters of natural law. The S. Congregation for the Doctrine of the Faith, however, in its *The Instruction on the Ecclesial Vocation of the Theologian* (May 4, 1990): n.16, says, "By reason of the connection between the orders of creation and redemption and by reason of the necessity, in view of salvation, of knowing and observing the whole moral law, the competence of the Magisterium also extends to that which concerns natural law."

7. On relativism, see *Veritatis Splendor*, n. 54; on proportionalism, n. 75.

8. This notion, first put forward by Herbert Doms, *The Meaning of Marriage* (New York: Sheed Ward, 1939), Chapter IX, "The Relative Importance of the Purposes of Marriage," pp. 83-97 and rejected by Pius XII (*Decretum de finibus matrimonii*, April 1, 1944), was argued from a historical point of view by John T. Noonan, Jr., *Contraception: A History of its Treatment by Catholic Theologians and Canonists* (Cambridge: Belknap, Harvard University Press, 1965). Vatican II in *Gaudium et Spes*, however, continued to teach that "by their very nature, the institution of matrimony itself and conjugal love are ordained for the procreation and education of children, and find in them their ultimate crown." The Council and *Humanae Vitae* avoided the traditional terms "primary" and "secondary ends" to correct misinterpretations that married love is merely a means to procreation and to show that although the couple's

love is an end in itself (a *bonum honestum*, not a *bonum utile*) it is an end ordered to the further end of procreation. If our species did not need to procreate, would we be divided into male and female? Marital love is a particular kind of human friendship *specified* as sexual, i.e., between man and woman as such and therefore procreative. On this question see the still valuable article of John C. Ford, S.J., "Marriage: Its Meaning and Purpose," *Theological Studies*, 3 (1942): 333-374.

9. A. Kosnick, et al., *Human Sexuality: New Directions in American Catholic Thought. A Study Commissioned by the Catholic Theological Society of America* (New York: Paulist, 1977). This report was promptly criticized by the Magisterium but the opinions it expressed still have advocates in the Church nearly twenty years later.

10. Noonan, in the work already cited, traces this history in great detail.

11. For the history of this see G. E. Joyce, S.J., *Christian Marriage: An Historical and Doctrinal Study* (New York: Sheed and Ward, 1933); Edward Schillebeeckx, O.P., *Marriage: Human Reality and Saving Mystery*, 2 vols. in one (New York: Sheed and Ward, 1965).

12. On the early origins of priestly celibacy, see Christian Cochini, S.J., *Apostolic Origins of Priestly Celibacy* (San Francisco: Ignatius Press, 1990) and Roman Cholij, *Clerical Celibacy in East and West* (Burgess Street Leominster, Herefordshire: Fowler and Wright Books, 1989).

13. The revised NAB translates the vivid Greek for teachers "who tickle the ear" (*didaskaloi kethomenoi ten akoen*) as ones who appeal to "insatiable curiosity."

Chapter 8

MORAL RELATIVISM
AND THE NEW *CATECHISM*

Ralph McInerny, Ph. D.

Pope John Paul II tells us at the outset of *Veritatis Splendor* (no. 5) that the encyclical was delayed so that the new *Catechism* might first appear. This order of appearance was not observed for American readers, however, and thus it would have been pardonable if an American reader thought that the second part of the *Catechism* took its cue from the encyclical rather than vice versa.

Part Two of the *Catechism* is concerned with Christian morality. The encyclical, noting that a series of magisterial documents had previously dealt with particular moral questions, sought to lay out the great context of the Christian life and its teleology. Unlike the *Catechism*, the encyclical has the special aim of showing how the foundations of Christian morality are jeopardized by the teaching of some moral theologians. "It is no longer a matter of limited and occasional dissent, but of an overall and systematic calling into question of traditional moral doctrine, on the basis of certain anthropological and ethical presuppositions" (no. 4). What the dissent of moral theologians has done is to muddle the very notion of intrinsically evil acts.

This recognition makes any discussion of moral relativism far more complicated than it had hitherto seemed. Once it was possible to see the faith and the magisterium as the one remaining bulwark and reminder of the once commonplace recognition that there are certain acts that one may never licitly do. On that basis, a discussion of relativism might seem to involve a disagreement between those who had the inestimable advantage of divine faith to bolster their grasp of moral facts and those who had not. Indeed it looked as if men, left to their own devices, inevitably lose awareness of even the most fundamental moral truths. *Veritatis Splendor*—and the quarter of a century of theological dissent which called it forth—makes inescapable the realization that the discussion is intramural as well.

Cardinal Newman, in an essay included in *The Idea of a University* called "On a Form of infidelity of the day," contrasted the 19th century with the medieval period. In the Middle Ages, he observed, foes of the faith were found within the walls, and this made discernment of error difficult. In the 19th century, the foes of Christianity are conveniently arrayed against her across a chasm of disbelief. The conflict, Newman thought, had thereby become clearer.

In Newman's terms, we now have the worst of two worlds. Not only is there a militant moral relativism outside the Church, and one which has an increasing formative effect on our culture, but there is moral relativism parading as a legitimate expression of Christian, indeed of Catholic, morality.

My remarks will accordingly be divided into two major parts. First, I will say something of the sources of secular moral relativism. Second, I will discuss the attack on intrinsically evil acts by some Catholic moral theologians. It will emerge that the latter owe a good deal to the former.

1. Secular Moral Relativism

Before I begin, I want to take into account an obvious objection. Someone might plausibly say that, far from being one of moral relativism, our age is rife with moral absolutes. Everywhere one turns, one hears certain modes of conduct unequivocally condemned as always and everywhere wrong. It is wrong to smoke, to pollute, to say where AIDS comes from, to use "he" and "man" as they have always been used by the great writers of English, and so on and on. These precepts might not look much like those of the Decalogue but they have the same exceptionless ring to them. Moral relativism indeed.

The difficulty makes it clear that there are any number of candidates for the role of moral absolute. But what are the criteria of a moral rule being absolute? As soon as we pose this question, we see that the proposed moral absolutes are little more than assertions.

Never smoke. Why not? Because it is harmful to your health. So what? If my body is my own, to do with as I wish, I can decide to smoke to a fare-thee-well. The culture in which Smoke Free has become a crusaders slogan deprives the New Puritans of any rational basis for their dislike. Abortion is now so embedded in the culture as a right which is founded simply on the freedom of the autonomous individual that the prohibition of smoking is soon revealed as a tyrannical imposition of an arbitrary standard on others. After all, those who object to abortion are taken to be voicing a merely private sentiment. Smoking may be suicidal, but there is a right to commit suicide, is there not?

I am suggesting that putative moral absolutes turn out to be something altogether different when we examine the ethical underpinning of the culture in which they are asserted. Those ethical underpinnings are, if Alasdair MacIntrye is right, quite simply emotivism. We are all emotivists now, MacIntrye says; emotivism has become general in our culture. And what is emotivism?

In 1903, G. E. Moore published *Principia Ethica*, a book which gave new impetus to a puzzle first dwelt on by David Hume. Moral judgments take the form of precepts, of gerundives and imperatives, and they often show up as the conclusion of an argument whose premises are factual. This is the case and that is the case, therefore you

113

ought to do such and such. How can you derive an Ought from an Is, Hume wondered. G. E. Moore said you can't, and that to the attempt to do so constitutes a fallacy, the naturalistic fallacy.

Now this supposed fallacy consists in thinking that the way things are provides a basis for knowing what we ought to do. This is an astounding claim—what we are and what the world is have nothing whatsoever to do with judgments of moral good and evil! How then are we to understand such remarks as "It would be wrong for you to do that" or "For you to do this would be morally good"? Moore himself had two replies. One was that goodness is a simple nonnatural property that we intuit in the way in which we perceive colors. Either you see yellow or you don't, and the same is true of moral values. This theory was called Intuitionism. It has the obvious defect of not accounting for the way moral claims are disputed, argued for, etc.

Moore elsewhere embraced Utilitarianism, the theory that employs as the criterion of action the greatest good of the greatest number. But this theory notoriously permits us to do what is generally considered to be evil in order to obtain the greatest good for the greatest number.

It is of course puzzling how an Intuitionist could have also held a theory that makes 'good' and 'bad' empirically calculable qualities of actions. In any case, in the sequel to Moore, attention was drawn to the nature of argument in moral philosophy, and room was made for the factual, for natural truths, in the moral order, but they gained entry in a quite controlled way. R. M. Hare provided perhaps the most elegant and extensive account of the way we reason about action. Given a principle as to what the good is, any number of observations about ourselves and the world would figure in the application of the principle. So interesting was Hare's account of the logic of moral language that he drew his own and others' attention away from the status of the principles themselves. Granted that we can argue from them; is there any way in which we can argue to or for them? That is, what if it is the principles rather than their application that is questioned? When Hare himself confronted this question, he revealed that his whole theory amounts to what I have called Postponed Emotivism.

The principles themselves are simply chosen. Why? They just are. But what if someone rejects those principles? Nice people don't. Hare quite literally thought this. He thought that only a fanatic would reject the rule of justice, for example. In calling the dissenter a fanatic, Hare might seem to be acquitting him of irrationality. Alas, this is not so. To underscore this, Hare actually puts "fanatic" in quotation marks, meaning that while you and I and our friends might regard the man who advocates genocide as unclubbable, we cannot say that he is wrong.

In short, the whole of ethics depends on principles we just happen to like, to find comfortable or familiar or whatever-- but which cannot in any significant sense be called true. Quite different principles could function in moral argument and they are every bit as good as ours. The relativism of the 20th century is thus rightly referred to as Emotivism, and it is surely not adventurous to say that Emotivism has become general. So general, that it has all but taken over legal and political theory.

When asked what the rule of law is, an influential and large number of theorists will say that it is the brokering of different points of view. Let us say that you and I are in dispute as to whether or not I can put up a billboard that effectively conceals your cathedral. You take me to court. Who is right and who is wrong? Neither of us. Your view is given the value of 1, my view is given the value of 1, and the task of the judge is to adjudicate our differences in such a way that there is no suggestion that your view is right and mine is wrong, or vice versa.

During the Iran-Contra hearings, it was regularly said that the genius of the American system is that it does not endorse any particular ethical or moral outlook. All moral outlooks are equal in our system. The system is simply the means whereby we permit citizens to have moral views without obstructing other citizens from having different and conflicting ones. The system itself is neutral.

Well, I have gone on enough about such familiar matters. From the Congress to the Op-ed page and letters to the editor, we are familiar with the response that any moral view in conflict with one's own is simply an expression of the other's feelings, and can lay no claim to be true and binding on others. The same is true of the view being attacked, of course. Moral judgments are expressions of feelings. As such, they can never rise to the dignity of being contradicted. If I say I have lower back pain and you say I don't, the two remarks are perfectly compatible. I am reporting on my back, you are reporting on yours. And so it has become with moral judgments. We may seem to be at odds, but we really aren't: you are reporting on your feelings, I am reporting on mine.

This is the situation that the Church faces in the wider society. This is what religious faith itself is taken to be, a personal quirk, an oddity of feeling, something private. Where the very notion of truth has been weakened, how will Christ be understood when He says, "I am the truth"?

I would not want to leave you with the notion that our situation is this: on the one hand, we have a moral relativism stemming from emotivism, on the other we have an objective morality, one which the faith both presupposes and strengthens. If one opts for emotivism or if one opts for a natural law ethic, this would then seem to be merely a choice unguided by the way things are. If that were our situation, we would in effect be adopting emotivism ourselves. If an objective morality is simply one we feel comfortable with, we are as much emotivists as the emotivists.

What has to be done, and I simply gesture toward the task now, is to show that emotivism is conceptually incoherent. It is not one among several reasonable positions—of course it would never describe itself that way—but on its own terms it is incoherent. One would go to the very heart of the project—the supposed neutral adjudication of substantive positions no one of which is to be endorsed as true. Underlying this brokering is the assumption that it is important to honor the rights of others to choose for themselves. It doesn't take a weekend in Dallas to realize that this is a substantive view about human agents. And it is one which, reflected on, makes it clear that not just any old choice can be fulfilling of the kind of agent we are.

It is not then just a matter of different strokes for different folks. The philosophical task is to show that no one can be a coherent emotivist, that to be an emotivist requires common substantive views about the human agent and his choices, and that there must be criteria for appraising when such choices are made well and when they are not. In short, there is truth and falsity in morals because of the way we and the world are.

2. Relativism Within the Walls

From time immemorial, Jews and Christians and pagans have held that there are certain acts which no one can licitly do. The random slaughter of the innocent, lying, taking another's spouse, homosexual acts, stealing, and so on, are actions which in themselves, because of what they are, are wrong. In the phrase, they are intrinsically evil. They are not wrong because they lead to bad consequences, though usually they do. In their very nature they are wrong. They are absolutely wrong.

In *Veritatis Splendor*, summarizing the way in which Christianity answers the most fundamental question of human life—what must I do to be saved?—employing as the *Catechism* had done the story of the rich young man, John Paul II draws out from the account the way in which negative precepts protect and preserve the positive moral ideal. When told that he must keep the commandments—and Jesus enumerates a number of them—the young man replies that he already does. Jesus then tells him what he must do if he would be perfect. The Holy Father draws out the significance of this sequence. The negative precepts, thou shalt nots, do not of course exhaust the moral life, let alone the Christian life. Rather, they exclude acts which can never be morally good. Observing such precepts releases one for the positive pursuit of the good, which is so various and infinitely imitable that no two good human persons will be identical. If that is true of the natural order, it is true *a fortiori* of the supernatural. In imitating Christ, the saints differentiate themselves from one another, but in a perfectly compatible way.

Since negative precepts, the recognition that some acts are intrinsically evil, play such an important role in establishing the limits of moral discourse, any weakening of our sense of intrinsic evil will have devastating effects on morality. But it is just this weakening that the Pope sees as the effect of over a quarter century of theological dissent. And *Veritatis Splendor* was written to make it crystal clear that the theological positions criticized are not valid expressions of Christian morality.

The *Catechism of the Catholic Church* has this to say about good and evil acts:

A *morally good* act requires the goodness of the object, of the end, and of the circumstances together. An evil end corrupts the action, even if the object is good in itself (such as praying and fasting "in order to be seen by men").

The *object of the choice* can by itself vitiate an act in its entirety. There are some concrete acts—such as fornication—that it is always wrong to choose, because choosing them entails a disorder of the will, that is, a moral evil. (no. 1755)

It is therefore an error to judge the morality of human acts by considering only the intention that inspires them or the circumstances (environment, social pressure, duress or emergency, etc.) which supply their context. There are acts which, in and of themselves, independently of circumstances and intentions, are always gravely illicit by reason of their object; such as blasphemy and perjury, murder and adultery. One may not do evil so that good may result from it. (no. 1756)

These passages from the *Catechism* invoke the three fonts of morality which figure so prominently in *Veritatis Splendor*. For most of us, they recall the *Prima Secundae* of St Thomas Aquinas's *Summa theologiae*, particularly questions 18, 19 and 20, three of the longest questions in the whole *Summa*. In what has gone before, Thomas has discussed at great length man's ultimate end and then gone into an extraordinary analysis of the structure of human action. The discussion of end provides the definition of the moral part of the *Summa*. In those opening five questions, Thomas magisterially relates the imperfect attainment of the end possible in this life with the perfect attainment of it possibly only *in patria*. This enabled him to relate the Aristotelian discussion in the *Nicomachean Ethics* with Christian revelation and to exhibit the complementarity rather than the opposition of natural morality and Christian morality. As mentioned earlier, this recognition is a hallmark of Church moral teaching. As human beings, we all, Christian and non-Christian, have the inborn capacity to discern good and evil. The human agent is ordered to the good; there is never any need to persuade a human being that he ought to do what is good for him to do. Augustine saw in this natural impulse toward the good a hunger for God, for goodness itself. "You have made us for yourself, O Lord..." Similarly, Chesterton once remarked that the young man knocking on the brothel door is looking for God.

He has the wrong address, to be sure, but his is a misdirected desire for the good.

It is reason that must guide this desire for the good, reason which formulates precepts and guidelines which enable us to avoid the merely apparent good and to seek the true good. The inborn capacity to discern good and evil gives rise straightaway to some precepts which, like "Do good and avoid evil" articulate the very nature of human action. These first, most common, and inescapably true precepts are called natural law. It is among such precepts that are found those negative precepts which express kinds of action we may never licitly do. Independently of personal and cultural and temporal differences, there are certain types of act which we are always and everywhere forbidden to do.

I said earlier that there is no shortage in our times of moral absolutes, that is, of prohibitions to act which admit of no exceptions. I also suggested that the regnant moral theory reduces these to mere assertions of feeling, of subjective attitude. What are the criteria for a moral absolute's truly being a moral absolute?

An exceptionless precept is clearly one that is understood to apply to all men because of what human agents are. Any kind of conduct that would always and everywhere thwart the human good is for that very reason always and everywhere forbidden to each and every human agent. This involves the judgment that a certain kind of act is indeed incompatible with what the human agent is—and I mean as agent. Man is not born inert and then begins to desire. We are appetites, desires, inclinations. A *nature* is a principle of activity, the seat of the desire for the fulfillment of the one having that nature. Above all we are endowed with a will, with rational appetite, which has as its object our complete good. The direction of appetite and of will by mind implies a grasp of what we are, of what truly is fulfilling of us and of what truly is thwarting of us. Again, it is the absence of such a basis in truth that undercuts most latter day moral absolutes. If each of us is what he chooses to make himself, there is nothing easier than simply declaring a precept inapplicable—and the denial is as true as the affirmation, that is, not true at all.

A word on the so-called Naturalistic Fallacy, the supposed flaw in moving from Is to Ought. This difficulty can only arise if we think that descriptions are of inert and undirected objects such that one is seeking to bring about a first choice, a first desire, a first action. No classical philosopher could have imagined such a fallacy. We become aware of ourselves as drawn to, attracted by, any number of things, and overarching in all such particular appetites is the will's desire for our complete good as grasped by reason. This desire is not consequent on any decision on our part. It is what we are. Practical discourse, accordingly, is not a matter of starting a process, but of directing it. The fallacy behind the Naturalistic Fallacy has a lot more to do with the Is than with the Ought.

The precepts of Natural Law are reason's guidance in our pursuit of goods to which we already naturally tend. We do not choose to seek to preserve ourselves in existence, we do not choose to hunger and thirst, we do not choose to be attracted to the opposite sex, we did not choose to live in a community—we are born into one and would not survive if we were not nurtured and cared for over a long span of time by our parents—we do not choose to want to know. These inclinations are not natural law precepts of course. A natural law precept is reason's judgment that the goods of these inclinations must be pursued in such a way that the complete good of the person is achieved—and that complete good is communal.

Presupposed by such precepts is the fact that we are free and intelligent agents, that our acts are voluntary and that we are answerable for them, responsible. "Why did you do that?" is a question which, when it is relevant, makes it clear that we are dealing with moral action. When we are asked why we are growing old or going bald or the like, we can give causes, but the causes are not choices and decisions of ours. The moral "Why" bears on those activities which we freely and knowingly bring about.

What is the answer to that "Why?"

As both the *Catechism* and *Veritatis Splendor* make clear, there are three possible answers. Answers like: Because I wanted to spare you pain. Or: Because there were children in the room.

But these answers presuppose a more fundamental one, that bearing on what precisely it was that we did. The previous answers cite some further end we had in view, or the circumstances in which we found ourselves. But such answers are parasitic on what precisely it was we did, the object of the act.

Object, end and circumstances. As the *Catechism* points out: "The object, the intention, and the circumstances make up the three 'sources' of the morality of human acts" (no. 1757). Furthermore, "A morally good act requires the goodness of its object, of its end, and of its circumstances together" (no.1760). Again, "The object chosen morally specifies the act of willing accordingly as reason recognizes and judges it good or evil" (no. 1758).

And then: "There are concrete acts that it is always wrong to choose, because their choice entails a disorder of the will, i.e., a moral evil. One may not do evil so that good may result from it" (no. 1761).

In short, the *Catechism* states the same doctrine as *Veritatis Splendor* and both are simply restating the traditional moral teaching of the Church, beautifully codified by Thomas Aquinas, but by no means original with him. If Thomas Aquinas figures prominently both in the *Catechism* and in the Encyclical, this is because, as Leo XIII said in *Aeterni Patris*, in reading Thomas we seem to be reading all of the Fathers at once.

The theological dissent to which *Veritatis Splendor* devotes so much of Chapter Two is taken to have embraced some version of the view that one may do evil in order that good may come of it. This is why the position criticized is variously called Teleologism and Consequentialism. It is linked with the notion of a Fundamental Option, that is, with the notion that there is an orientation to the good so profound and basic that it cannot be disturbed by single acts which have traditionally been judged intrinsically evil.

What we have heard for more than a quarter of a century are moral theologians who have devised ways for speaking of masturbation, fornication, adultery, homosexual acts and abortion as not always and everywhere destructive of the good. Nor are these discussions of the imputability of guilt. They have to do with the very nature of the acts in question.

The passages from the *Catechism* just cited state that the object of the act—e.g., lying with another's spouse—is objectively disordered, and no intention of some beneficial consequence can ever justify it. Dissenting moral theologians are taken to waffle on this.

Have they? Father Richard McCormick in a recent article in *Theological Studies* surveyed first reactions to *Veritatis Splendor* and, clearly considering himself one of the theologians being censored, vehemently denied that either he or any of his fellows had ever said that it is sometimes morally okay to perform an intrinsically evil act. This is a disingenuous response.

Of course Father McCormick never said that it is sometimes morally okay to do something which it is never morally okay to do. But has he ever said that when the object of the act is disordered it is possible to do it because of one's intention?

Yes and no.

As is clear, the moral tradition in which Father McCormick was raised and which in his early writings he accepted, as did Joseph Fuchs and others he defends against the accusations of *Veritatis Splendor*—the moral tradition all these men know, distinguishes object, end, and circumstances. It holds that, in order to be good, an act must have a good object, a good intention, and be performed in appropriate circumstances. A good intention cannot trump a bad object, but a good object can be vitiated by a bad intention or because the circumstances are inappropriate.

Father McCormick now wishes to distinguish motive—the end—and intention, which bears on the object. Now this is all well and good, even traditional; Thomas calls the object the proximate end and the further purpose the remote end of the act. But what is this insistence on intention supposed to do? In Father McCormick's hands, it radically alters what is meant by the object of the act.

Until I know the person's intention, he and other heterodox moral theologians assert, I do not know whether sleeping with another's spouse constitutes a disordered object and amounts to an act of adultery. Until I know a person's intention in manipulating his genitalia for purposes of pleasure, I do not know whether it is an instance of masturbation.

But this simply smuggles into the object, the remote end and suggests that until we know what the agent has in mind in doing X, we cannot say that X is disordered. I call this defense disingenuous because Father McCormick, who was trained in the traditional moral theology, knows what he is doing. He is redefining the object of the act, including in it the purpose of the agent, and suggesting that what is done, the object in the traditional sense, is morally neutral until we know the agent's intention.

This is not, I repeat, a discussion of the imputability of guilt, but of the nature of the act done.

What is being condemned in *Veritatis Splendor* is the claim that "lying with another's spouse," when this is the object of a voluntary act, is insufficient for us to decide whether it is an intrinsically evil act.

That such prestidigitation with the terms of the discussion should be accompanied by an unworthy imputation of some kind of sexual prudery to the Magisterium no longer, I suppose, surprises. It has become *de rigueur* for theologians to speak ill of the Pope and the Magisterium. Father McCormick makes the impudent accusation that the Church employs one notion of object of an act in speaking of sexual morality and quite another when speaking of other moral questions. That is, the teaching office of the Roman Catholic Church is engaged in duplicity for ideological reasons having to do with repressed sexuality. He actually suggests that the Magisterium regards the physical act as such as the object of the moral act. Killing a human being can be described as simply a natural occurrence such that the same account would cover both murder and self-defense. Father McCormick actually suggests that the Magisterium regards "A having intercourse with B" as the object of the act when sexual morality is under discussion. Since this would prevent any distinction between conjugal acts and adultery, a distinction the Magisterium is known to make, Father McCormick is guilty of a shameful derogation of the teaching office of the Church. He knows that what constitutes the intrinsically disordered object of an act is "A's having intercourse with B's spouse."

What in the name of God, we may well ask ourselves, motivated moral theologians to abandon the traditional morality and at least seemingly to be ready and willing to negotiate away every traditionally recognized, and biblically based, moral absolute? It is of course undeniable that the atmosphere created by the moral teaching of many moral theologians suggested that the old prohibitions against masturbation, fornication, adultery, homosexual acts, etc., must be rethought and that, when they are, it turns out that such deeds are not always wrong. Over the past quarter of century, magisterial documents have dealt with one or more of these efforts to redefine Christian morality. Now with the *Catechism* and *Veritatis Splendor* they are indelibly characterized as false doctrines.

Dissenting moral theologians have got themselves into this heterodox corner for two reasons. First, an uncritical acceptance of the zeitgeist. Misinterpreting John XXIII's remarks at the opening of the Council to mean that traditional doctrine was to be pitched out of those opened windows as contemporary moral theory rushed in, they have been influenced by moral theories which, since they are philosophically flawed, are dubious instruments of moral theology.

Second, they were moved by false compassion. One does not have to live long to see what messes we make of our lives, and to see that for most the mess is mixed up with sexuality. The sensate culture in which we live, with its sick emphasis on sex as mere sensation, affects us all. The ideal of chastity, if preached at all nowadays, is preached on a consequentialist basis. The difficulties of pastoral care in these circumstances are enormous. What to do? Perhaps if the prohibitions were less stringent, more flexible...

Underlying this, I think, is the view, incredible in a moralist, that immorality can be fulfilling of the human agent. That a little bit of it might be beneficial. Waive the ban on contraception, say, and families and spouses would flourish. Of course, the moral theologian did not want to say it is sometimes good to be bad. Rather, he set about redefining badness. If only we redefine the intrinsically evil, and thus let people do what remains intrinsically evil despite our definition, then things will go better with them, with their families, with society. Well, *circumspice*; on a consequentialist basis, consequentialism has failed.

The rich young man of the Gospel, having kept the commandments, did not want to make the next step for which his observance had prepared him. To keep the commandments is already to lead the good life. The commandments consist of negative and positive precepts. One of the beauties of the *Catechism* is the way in which its discussions of the Commandments, *seriatim*, draws attention to the moral ideal, the Christian ideal, that good which is the inexhaustible end of all our aspirations. The prohibitions do not thwart the human agent. It is the acts they prohibit which thwart and stunt and render us less than human. There is a logic to the good life, which draws us onward; there is also a logic of evil which seeks ever more disordered chaos, making it more and more difficult for us to turn back.

124

The misguided efforts of moral theologians to issue passes to the morally confused have caused incalculable harm, in the Church, in pastoral work, in the lives of Catholics. Armed with the *Catechism*, the catechism of Vatican II, and *Veritatis Splendor*, and that long series of perceptive, wise and truly pastoral magisterial documents, we can begin to repair the damage.

Chapter 9

WOMEN AND HEALTH CARE: A CATHOLIC PERSPECTIVE

E. Joanne Angelo, M.D.

Certain Health Care issues are of special interest to women because they deal with diseases which affect women in a particular manner (women's *health*). Other health related issues are of a special concern to women because they tap into women's caring concern for others (*care*). "Women not only define themselves in a context of human relationships but also judge themselves in terms of their ability to care," Carol Gilligan asserts in her landmark book on feminine psychology, *In a Different Voice*, published in 1982.[1]

This presentation will address some of the most salient *health* issues for women and then consider the *care* of children, the elderly and terminally ill which has been perennially a woman's concern.

Childbearing

Childbearing is exclusively a woman's prerogative. "The history of every human being passes through the threshold of a woman's motherhood," the Holy Father reminds us in his apostolic letter of the *Dignity and Vocation of Women.*[2] "The moral and spiritual strength of a woman is joined to her awareness that God entrusts the human being to her in a special way," he concludes.[3]

A woman is aware that a tiny human person has been entrusted to her as soon as she realizes that she is pregnant. She looks to the health care system to provide the best prenatal care possible for herself and for her developing child.

In the current health care debate economic factors have taken on disproportionate significance. The long-standing public health argument that good prenatal care produces cost-savings because it reduces the costs of medical complications associated with low birth weight infants has recently been challenged. Although the scientific certainty of the cost-savings argument for prenatal care may be difficult to prove, it is important that these programs be adequately funded and made available to all women from the beginning of their pregnancies. The authors of a recent *New England Journal of Medicine* article on this topic conclude:

> We should recognize that measuring the costs and benefits of any treatment is neither simple nor straightforward. It is very possible that prenatal care is beneficial in less easily measured ways—for example, by producing healthier and happier pregnancies and promoting better relationships with health care providers. These, in turn, may encourage better parenting, more complete childhood immunization, and improvements in other health related behavior....'many things that really count cannot be counted.'...It may be better to ask not, 'How much does it save?' but rather, 'How much is it worth?'[4]

128

Prenatal care is worth a great deal more than is currently being allocated to it, and yet we hear of government proposals to reduce funding for these programs even in the face of a shamefully high infant mortality rate in our country. At 8.5 deaths for every 1000 live births, the United States ranked 24th in infant mortality among comparable countries in 1992 (the last year for which statistics are available).[5]

Women experiencing untimely pregnancies have needs which go beyond excellence in medical care. They need to be surrounded by a network of supportive services including counseling, housing, financial, educational and employment resources, and adoption services. Many of these services are generously supplied by Catholic hospitals and agencies at present, but the need outweighs the supply, especially in the face of threatened government cuts in programs to aid unwed mothers. More services and better outreach are needed to inform women with untimely pregnancies of the very real alternatives to abortion which are available to them, often without charge.

Women who have suffered the tragedy of rape or sexual abuse require specialized services to help them cope with the trauma they have experienced. Even in the rare event of pregnancies in these cases, the outcome need not be negative. The fiancé of a young woman who became pregnant as a consequence of rape told me that on Christmas eve, looking at St. Joseph in the crèche scene, he realized that Joseph did not know what had happened to Mary but he took her in and cared for her. This heroic young man felt that he could not do anything less. He offered to marry her right away, but she declined until after the baby was born. As soon as was legally possible after their wedding, he adopted her baby daughter.

Catholic hospitals should reach out to victims of rape and sexual abuse with compassion and offer them counseling and medical care consistent with Catholic medical-moral principles. It would be tragic if women in these circumstances were to avoid the Catholic Health Care System out of shame, or because they believed that their health care needs would not be addressed with kindness and compassion in a timely and effective manner.

Interruption of Pregnancy

If the very special relationship between a pregnant woman and the developing child within her is interrupted prematurely, a number of negative sequelae occur. This is true whether the interruption of pregnancy is due to miscarriage, tubal pregnancy, stillbirth, or induced abortion.

For example, the incidence of breast cancer is increased in young women whose first pregnancy is interrupted at an early stage. It is believed that the rapidly proliferating breast cells, destined to differentiate into lactating cells at term, are left to proliferate in a relatively undifferentiated state if the pregnancy is interrupted, and may, therefore, become malignant over time. However because breast cancer may take ten years to develop, the actual malignancy may not be diagnosed until years later.[6, 7, 8] Oral contraceptives have also been associated with a higher risk of breast cancer and cervical cancer in young women who have taken the pill early in their reproductive lives. Many oral contraceptives cause the destruction of an already established pregnancy by altering the hormonal environment at the time of implantation.[9]

A mother's grief following the death of her child before the child's expected day of birth, or following a premature delivery is well documented in the medical literature. A recent review article in the *American Journal of Psychiatry* listed 90 references on this topic.[10] Obstetrical hospitals have developed teams of nurses, doctors and social workers who help parents cope with the loss of their children in the perinatal period by encouraging them to see, hold and name their dead baby, take photographs, and arrange a funeral service and burial. The medical literature acknowledges that *very early* pregnancy loss due to miscarriage or ectopic pregnancy is more difficult to resolve because there is no body to identify, no child to name or bury, nothing concrete to mourn. The ninety references in the *American Journal of Psychiatry* article on perinatal grief, however, include only one reference to grief after induced abortion—a reference to a book by the same author in which he presumes that, because a woman chose to have an abortion, she would not grieve the loss of her child.[11]

Abortion

Abortion *is* followed by a profound grief reaction in many women. These women typically find themselves alone and unsupported in their grieving. Abortion clinics provide no perinatal grief team to assist a post-abortion woman. She has no child to hold or to name, no photographs, no wake or funeral, no grave to visit, no memories. She must cope not only with the loss of the child she will never know, but also with her personal responsibility in the child's death with its ensuing guilt and shame.

The post-abortion woman may have difficulty understanding her ambivalent feelings—on the one hand, relief that she is no longer pregnant (a feeling that is often short-lived), and a profound sense of loss and emptiness on the other. The defensive denial of her tender and protective feelings toward her baby which made it possible for her to engage an abortionist to destroy her child lasts usually for at least a short time after the procedure. This may explain why exit interviews with women leaving abortion clinics usually find them to be relieved and apparently guilt free.

Feelings of loss, profound sadness and guilt may threaten to overwhelm a woman in the weeks and months after an abortion. Society offers her no assistance in the mourning. She is expected to be grateful that "her problem is solved," and to "get on with her life" as though nothing significant had happened. Yet, she is poignantly aware of the date her child would have been born. Reminders continue to threaten her defensive denial and repression in subsequent months and years. —anniversaries of her abortion, other children of the age her child would have been, Mother's Day, the omni-present abortion debate in the media, a visit to the gynecologist, the sound of a suction machine in the dentist's office, or the sound of a vacuum cleaner at home, a baby in a television ad, a new birth, another death in the family, a pro-life homily. Any of these reminders may trigger a sudden flood of grief and despair, which, in turn, calls forth even more intense defensive responses and coping strategies.

A Pathological Grief Reaction often ensues which can include a variety of physical symptoms which mimic various medical conditions. After an abortion a woman may turn to alcohol or drugs to get to sleep and to avoid the recurring nightmares and the intrusive thoughts which haunt her day and night: "I killed my baby! I killed my baby! I don't deserve to live!" Flashbacks to the abortion experience often occur without warning. She may throw herself into intense activity—work, study, or recreation, or attempting to deal with her feelings of loneliness and emptiness by binge eating alternating with purging or anorexia. She may make intense efforts to repair intimate relationships or develop new ones inappropriately, becoming sexually promiscuous and putting herself at risk for sexually transmitted diseases and recurring pregnancies. Complaints of vague abdominal pain, sexual dysfunction, and infertility may cause her to seek medical treatment from one physician after another, and the very examinations to which she is subjected may cause flashbacks to the abortion experience resulting in extreme anxiety for her and for her physicians. Discouragement, despair, clinical depression, and suicide attempts often follow.[12, 13]

Reports in the medical literature have begun to document some of the medical and surgical complications of abortion: 240 women are reported to have died as a consequence of legal, induced abortion between 1972 and 1987 in the United States; uterine ruptures, sepsis, ectopic pregnancy, infertility and increased incidence of breast and cervical cancer are documented as linked to abortion.[14, 15] However, the lack of well-designed longitudinal studies have obscured the long term negative psychological effects of abortion on women and their families.

In a state of prolonged pathological grief, women are incapable of forming and sustaining stable spousal relationships, and of caring appropriately for subsequent children. They may have difficulty bonding with a new baby, or, conversely, become overprotective and inappropriately attached to the next child who bears the burden of replacing the aborted baby. Subsequent children may be at risk for the development of separation anxiety or for physical abuse.[16] Couples may be treated for infertility or dysfunctional marriages which are the result of abortion. Substance abuse, "burn out" on the job, psychosomatic symptoms, eating disorders, chronic depression, and suicide attempts which bring women to seek psychiatric care can often be traced to an abortion experience several years previously by means of a careful and complete history. Too often, however, only the presenting symptoms are treated. This may be due to physicians' lack of understanding of the significance of the abortion history coupled with health insurance payments which only focus on diagnosis related short term interventions.

In 1973 the *Journal of the National Medical Association* urged for systematic follow up of all abortion patients because, "the epidemiologic consequences of abortion may become statistically relevant in the not-too-distant future with far-reaching public health significance."[17] Over 30 million abortions have been performed in the United States since that time; the elective abortion is currently the most frequently performed operation in this country. The adverse sequelae of induced abortion constitute a risk of epidemic proportion to the public health, and to women's health in particular. Abortion has no place in Health Care as it represents neither *Health* nor *Care*. Pregnancy is not a disease, and its forced interruption is neither healthful nor caring either for the child who is destroyed or for the mother who may be burdened with the negative aftermath of abortion for the rest of her life.

Education in a Christian view of the family and of human sexuality which is integrated into all levels of instruction in our schools and catechetical programs is sorely needed in order to stem the tide of sexual promiscuity and abnormal sexual practices which result in untimely pregnancies and sexually transmitted diseases.

For example, *The Catechism of the Catholic Church* teaches:

> "Being man" or "being woman" is a reality which is good and willed by God... Man and woman are both with one and the same dignity "in the image of God." In their "being man" and "being woman," they reflect the Creator's wisdom and goodness... Man and woman were "made for each other"... In marriage God unites them in such a way that, by forming "one flesh," they can transmit human life: "Be fruitful and multiply and fill the earth." By transmitting human life to their descendants, man and woman as spouses cooperate in a unique way in the Creator's work.[18]

For example, *True Love Waits*, a program of the National Federation for Catholic Youth Ministry, promotes healthy lifestyles among adolescents—specifically the advancement of chastity—while at the same time assuring them that God understands better than any human being the difficulties and powerful urges with which they are dealing.

The supportive love of God, reflected in the life of Jesus, reassures us that even when we are weak and fail, the Lord's compassion and forgiveness are always there.[19]

Fertility and Infertility

Contraception and Natural Family Planning

The prescription of contraception for women of childbearing age has become common medical practice. Birth control pills represent the single most expensive category of drugs ordered by physicians in the Health Maintenance Organization to which I belong. Oral contraceptives are responsible for an annual expenditure of $2,000,000 in this particular H.M.O. (Tufts Health Plan), which is one of several in the Greater Boston area. This sum does *not* include the cost of other forms of contraception–diaphragms, cervical caps, IUDs, Norplant implants, Depo-Provera injections and "all standard forms of male and female sterilization" which are also covered by the plan. Side effects of birthcontrol pills are minimized by the H.M.O.'s communications to physicians, although we are cautioned about the increased incidence of strokes, heart attacks and pulmonary emboli in young oral contraceptive users who are also smokers–problems which are rare in young women who are not on "the pill."[20] Recent reports of the incidence of breast cancer and cancer of the cervix with oral contraceptive use[21] are not mentioned. The cost of treatment of AIDS and other sexually transmitted diseases for which contraceptive users are at increased risk is not factored into this analysis, nor is the cost of abortions which often follow when the predicted 6% failure rate of oral contraception occurs. Even if the psychological toll of contraception and sterilization on women is ignored (and that of abortion when contraception fails), economics alone would mitigate against these practices being included among health services for women.

Let us return to Carol Gilligan's view that women define themselves in a context of human relationship and judge themselves in terms of their ability to care. Sexual intercourse, the most intimate of human relationships (except perhaps that of bearing a child) represents, for a woman, an occasion of giving herself totally and unconditionally to a man and being accepted reciprocally by him. Contraceptive intercourse which is pleasure-seeking or self-seeking, leaves her feeling empty, lonely, used and tossed aside. The gift of herself which she has offered has been rejected as has her wish to accept and care for her partner in a permanent relationship.[22] Small wonder that half of the marriages in our country end in divorce, and that the incidence of depression seems to be reaching epidemic proportions especially among women.[23] The words of John Paul II in Washington D.C. in 1979 may have been prophetic: "The great danger for family life in the midst of any society whose idols are pleasure, comfort and independence, lies in the fact that people close their hearts and become selfish. The fear of making permanent commitments can change the mutual love of husband and wife into two loves of self— two loves existing side by side, until they end in separation."[24]

In contrast to self-seeking contraceptive relationships, programs of Natural Family Planning, used either to space offspring in cases of serious need or to enhance conception, can help couples truly know one another, and express tenderness in selfless ways. "These methods respect the bodies of the spouses, encourage tenderness between them, and favor the education of an authentic freedom," as we read in the *Catechism of the Catholic Church.*[25] Dr. Thomas Hilgers at the Pope Paul VI Institute in Omaha has done a great deal to refine this method and teach it to physicians, nurses, and couples from a wide geographical area. The *British Medical Journal* recently published an article in favor of Natural Family Planning which described the method in considerable detail and reviewed large-scale studies of its effectiveness world wide. Unplanned pregnancy rates ranged from 0.2% to 3.6% (in contrast to Birth Control Pills' 6% failure rate). The article concludes "It is therefore important that the misconception that Catholicism is synonymous with ineffective birth control is laid to rest."[26] Of course, we know that Natural Family Planning is not "Catholic Birth Control" because the nature of human sexuality is not violated by it; however, it is clear that the effectiveness of the method in predicting fertile periods in women is now medically proven. Yet, too many Catholic physicians are unacquainted with natural methods of regulating births or dismiss N.F.P. because of misinformation about the method. Catholic Hospitals and dioceses would do well to promote education of health care professionals in Natural Family Planning and to establish readily available educational programs for couples who believe they need to space the births of their children or who are seeking assistance in conceiving.

Infertility

An increasing number of married couples are seeking infertility treatment while the number of babies available for adoption is decreasing. One out of every six couples (3-4 million couples) in the United States is now thought to be infertile. Male infertility accounts for 20-30%, female infertility accounts for 40-50%, and combined or unknown factors account for the remainder. The majority of women who are infertile are thought to be so because of scarring from abortions, sexually transmitted disease, or contraceptive devices.[27] Single women, some of whom are living in lesbian relationships, also seek the assistance of new reproductive technologies in order to become pregnant. The list of techniques and procedures in the field of reproductive health care is burgeoning: artificial insemination by spouse or donor, in vitro fertilization, cryopreservation of sperm in sperm banks, ovum donation, techniques for predetermining the sex of the fetus, selective abortion for sex selection or reduction of multiple pregnancies, surrogate motherhood, attempts at the development of artificial wombs, and "nursery environments" to maintain a fetus removed from the womb in the first trimester.

In the health care debate some say that an inordinate amount of money is spent for reproductive technologies which could be better spent elsewhere. A recent article in the *New England Journal of Medicine* places the cost of a single successful delivery with in vitro fertilization at from $67,00 to $800,000.[28] Some feminists hail these techniques as enhancing their reproductive freedom; others believe they represent the dehumanization of modern life, and the exploitation of women by a patriarchal health care system. An example of the latter viewpoint follows:

136

Feminist analysis guides us in rethinking the values that drive the search for new forms of reproductive technologies. It urges us to question the appropriateness of encouraging people to spend huge sums on creating certain sorts of children through IVF, and other forms of reproductive technology, while so many other children starve to death each year. IVF, like other forms of new reproductive technology, seems to strengthen, rather than weaken, social attitudes that underlie the politics of dominance and supremacy in our world.[29]

Diagnostic procedures and treatment techniques for infertility may be burdensome and immoral for both men and women. Semen samples are routinely collected through masturbation for diagnostic studies and for artificial insemination and in vitro fertilization. Women receive artificial hormone injections repeatedly to stimulate ovulation for IVF. Ovulation is monitored by means of frequent blood and urine samples and by ultrasound. Ova are removed by laparoscopy and combined with sperm in the laboratory. Some of the fertilized eggs are transferred to the uterus or fallopian tube, again by laparoscopy; the remainder may be frozen for later implantation or experimentation, or discarded (i.e., killed)

In vitro fertilization is successful in only 10 to 15% of cases selected as suitable. Each failed attempt is a huge disappointment for the woman and leaves her emotionally and physically exhausted. There is an increased incidence of ectopic pregnancy in women after IVF and other assisted conception procedures which is believed to be due not only to the underlying cause of infertility but also to adverse effects on egg and embryo quality due to induced ovulation and the altered hormonal environment created for the purpose of enhancing fertility.[30]

Even if pregnancy is achieved by means of new reproductive technology, and a healthy baby delivered, the result may be problematic for the mother. A mother of two sons, ages 12 and 11, came to me for the treatment of depression which had caused her to become immobilized and unable to care for her household and family. Her depression began precipitously one evening when she was saying good night to her eldest son. He asked her, "How come Peter (his brother) is so much like Daddy and I'm not?" Her son's words pierced her heart like a lance. This was the question she had been dreading for 12 years! Her first born son had been conceived by artificial insemination from an unknown donor, because she and her husband had been thought to be infertile. A year after the baby's birth she gave birth to another son—the product of normal sexual relations with her husband. She knew nothing about her eldest son's birth father. She struggled to compose herself and said, "Well, Peter is like Daddy on the outside, you're like Daddy on the inside." At her son's request she then came up with three personality characteristics which he shared with his father. She said, "Good night," went to her room, and threw herself across her bed, sobbing inconsolably.

The next day she called the physician who had performed the artificial insemination to ask for information about her son's birth father, and was told, "We didn't keep any records on donors, but I remember that he was a medical student—a handsome fellow. We used him several times. We used his brother too." She began to suspect that one any one of the doctors in town could be her son's father, and to be concerned that he would marry a half sister or other blood relative. She became obsessed with the question of whether or not to tell him how he was conceived. She would not have been consoled by an article in *Family Circle* magazine in supermarkets this fall which reported that a 35 year old engineer, who had been selling his sperm to a sperm bank weekly for fifteen years, was told that he had fathered more than 400 offspring. "I thought that was an enormous number," he said, "but they told me it was low for a popular donor— that others have produced over 1,000 children."[31]

Catholic women facing reproductive difficulties are bewildered and confused by the current state of the health care system with regard to the treatment of infertility, and uninformed about their ethical and moral significance. Catholic hospitals and medical schools cannot abandon this area because it is fraught with moral difficulties. Catholic physicians have considerable difficulty obtaining training in obstetrics and gynecology without participating in abortions and sterilizations and prescribing contraceptives and abortifacient drugs during their training years. They may not even be accepted into residency programs if it is known that they will object in conscience in these areas. Ob/Gyn residency programs are threatened with loss of accreditation if they fail to offer training in performing abortions.

Catholic medical schools and hospitals should strive for extraordinary excellence in their departments of Obstetrics and Gynecology and assume leadership in the development of new technologies which will enhance the health of mothers and their developing children from the moment of conception, and better diagnose and treat problems of infertility in accord with Catholic moral teaching. It may be possible to look to the expertise of medical school faculty from countries where anti-Catholic bias has not excluded them from state-of-the art training and research to assist us in this endeavor. Our Catholic medical institutions will then exemplify the Holy Father's teaching that, "there is no conflict between science and faith in the area of research and medical practices in the face of bioethical challenges, but rather a fruitful encounter, propitiated by the common aim of celebrating in man that life, which is God's gift."[32]

An important case report from St. George's Hospital Medical School in London is an example of how the newest reproductive technology can be employed in the service of life. The paper describes a normal term delivery after interuterine relocation of an ectopic pregnancy in an African woman. Early detection of the tubal pregnancy by means of sophisticated pregnancy tests and transvaginal ultrasound made intervention possible before tubal rupture. The pregnancy was surgically removed from the tube at laparotomy and carefully placed in the uterus through the cervix. The pregnancy was uneventful thereafter, and the mother delivered a healthy baby girl at 38 weeks by means of a spontaneous vaginal delivery.[33] Until very recently an ectopic pregnancy was thought to be non-viable, and ethical concern focused on appropriate surgical intervention for the removal of the potion of the damaged tube containing the fetus, the expected rupture of which would pose an emergent threat to the mother's life. Sophisticated early diagnostic tests and exquisitely delicate surgery have made it possible to save both the fetus' and the mother's life.

Issues of Aging

Issues of aging are of special interest to women because women can expect to live longer than men and are, therefore, at greater risk for the diseases of late life, such as osteoporosis, cardiovascular dis-

139

ease, and cancer. In addition, the care of elderly and terminally ill family members is of special concern to women.

Menopause, which used to be thought of as signaling the last stage of a woman's life, may soon mark her life's mid-point. After menopause, she can look forward to many productive and fulfilling years of "middle age," followed by a period now referred to as "young old," and finally, the "old old" time of her life. Her health in the post menopausal years is, to a certain extent, conditioned by patterns of health care, diet and exercise from childhood onward. Menopausal women receive varied medical advice about the advisability of hormone replacement therapy as treatment for menopausal symptoms, prevention of breast cancer and heart disease, and, in conjunction with calcium and vitamin D, as prevention of osteoporosis which can be very painful and even crippling in later years.

The National Institutes of Health has begun a number of longitudinal studies (the "Women's Health Initiative") which are being conducted simultaneously in 40 clinical centers across the nation. These research projects will involve 160,000 post-menopausal women in controlled studies of hormone replacement, dietary modifications (including calcium and vitamin D supplements and low fat diets), and an observational group in which women will report on their lifestyle habits, but not be asked to change them.[34] These studies, as well as other studies of women in their reproductive years, promise to yield a large database of health information about women. The present interest in research into women's health issues may provide an opportunity to include the collection of data about the long-term negative sequelae for women of abortion, sterilization and contraception—data which have been glaringly absent in most studies to date because researchers have failed to ask appropriate questions.

A woman who has spent her life caring for others may find herself alone late in life with no one to care for her. Small families, geographic separation of extended families, divorce, remarriage, and "blended families," have caused the disintegration of child-parent loyalties, and extended family networks. On the one hand, a middle aged woman may find herself sandwiched between her adult children who have come home to live and expect her to help with the care of the grandchildren while they work, and her own parents or grandparents who look to her for companionship and care. On the

140

other hand, she is likely to outlive her spouse by many years and to find herself widowed and alone late in life, with no apparent alternative other than to enter a nursing home where she fears that she will receive a minimal of custodial care in a dismal, impersonal, institutional environment for the last years of her life. Such a bleak outlook on the future, coupled with a fear of becoming a burden on family members whom they perceive as being poorly equipped to take care of them, may make women susceptible to arguments in favor of assisted suicide and euthanasia. In fact the "right to die" may be transformed for them into a perceived "need to die" or "duty to die."

However, this need not be so.

The Care of Frail and Terminally Ill Family Members

The final chapter of life's journey can be very beautiful. There are alternatives to impersonal institutional settings such as nursing homes or hospitals. I can attest to a shining example which is the Good Samaritan Hospice of the Archdiocese of Boston where I have been a psychiatric consultant for the past ten years. Hospice programs care for terminally ill patients at home or in home-like in-patient settings where they are surrounded by the affection of family and friends and compassionate staff whose primary role is not to *cure* them (because cure is no longer possible) but to *care* for them competently and charitably during the last months of their lives. Expert medical care is brought to the home or hospice facility by a team of specially trained nurses, physicians and home health aides. The patient and family are offered additional supportive service by social workers and volunteers. The hospice chaplain is available to provide pastoral care and sacramental ministry or to call in clergy of other faiths on request.

Those who would have us believe that death is necessarily accompanied by unbearable pain and suffering are just plain wrong! It is fear which typically motivates the terminally ill and their families to consider assisted suicide or euthanasia: fear of pain, fear of abandonment by those they love, fear of burdensome futile treatments, fear of loss of autonomy and personal dignity, and fear of becoming a burden on others. Compassionate health care (or better said, compassionate care of the whole person) such as that provided in a Christian hospice setting can enable patients to live out their lives with serenity and peace, surrounded by those they love until natural death occurs, thus making the notions of assisted suicide and euthanasia irrelevant.[35]

Home care of the chronically ill and frail elderly could be carried out following the same principles as hospice care if adequate funding were made available, so that similar services could be provided to those who wish to care for their loved ones within the family. Too often, at present, funding for long-term care is available only in institutional settings.

The compassionate care of the chronically ill and the dying until the last moment of natural life has an importance that extends far beyond the good of the individual and the family served. Our Holy Father told the Catholic health care leaders in Phoenix, "Your apostolate penetrates and transforms the very fabric of American society...As you alleviate suffering and seek to heal, you also bear witness to the Christian view of suffering and to the meaning of life and death as taught by your Christian faith."[36] "Suffering," he teaches elsewhere, "is present in the world in order to release love, in order to give birth to works of love toward neighbor, in order to transform the whole human civilization into a 'civilization of love'." [37]

Conclusion

In concluding this brief reflection on women and health care from a Catholic perspective I would like to consider the quotation with which Christina Hoff Sommers begins her recent book *Who Stole Feminism? How Women have Betrayed Women*:

> The New Feminism emphasizes the importance of 'the women's point of view', the Old Feminism believes in the primary importance of the human being.[38]

A contemporary Catholic view of women and health care incorporates both the view point of women regarding their own health issues, and women's concern for the primary importance and dignity of every human being.

Today one half of the students entering medical school are women. What a wonderful thing it would be for medicine if these women physicians of the future were to approach the provision of health care in a manner which truly conforms to their feminine nature! If they were to take Mary, the Mother of Mercy, as their model, to whom Jesus entrusts his church and all humanity as the Holy Father encourages us to do in the conclusion of *Veritatis Splendor.*[39]

Truly feminine Christian women physicians, nurses and other health care workers could transform our health care system into a shining example of a "work of love toward neighbor" which would help to transform our culture of death into the "civilization of love" which John Paul II foresees for our world in the third millennium.

Notes

1. Gilligan, Carol. *In A Different Voice* (Cambridge, MA: Harvard University Press, 1982), 17.

2. Pope John Paul II, *Mulieris Dignitatem*, no. 19.

3. Ibid., n. 30.

4. Huntington, Jane and Connell, Frederick A. "For every dollar spent—the cost savings argument for prenatal care." *NEJ Med* (1994): 331:1303-7.

5. Center for Disease Control and Prevention, Atlanta, GA. "Statistics re: infant mortality in the United States, 1992." *J Am Med Ass* (1995): 273:101.

6. Howe, H. L. et al. "Early abortions and breast cancer risk among women under age 40." *Int J Epidemiol* (1989): 18:300-304.

7. Olsson, H. et al. "Proliferation and DNA ploidy in malignant breast tumors in relation to early contraceptive use and early abortions." *Cancer* (1991): 67:1285-90.

8. Daling, Janet R. et al. "Risk of Breast Cancer Among Young Women: Relationship to induced Abortion." *J Natl Cancer Inst* (1994): 86:1584-92.

9. Chilvers, Clair. "Commentary: Oral contraceptives and cancer." *The Lancet* (1994): 344:1378-9.

10. Leon, Irving G. "The psychoanalytic conceptualization of perinatal loss: a multidimensional model." *Am J Psych* (1992):149:1461-72.

11. Leon, Irving G. *When A Baby Dies* (New Haven, Conn:Yale University Press, 1970), 63-65.

12. Angelo, E. Joanne. "Psychiatric sequelae of abortion: the many faces of post-abortion grief." *Linacre Quarterly* (1992): 59:69-80.

13. Angelo, E. Joanne. "The negative impact of abortion on women and families" in *Post-Abortion Aftermath: A Comprehensive Consideration,* ed. by Michael T. Mannion (Kansas City, MO: Sheed and Ward, 1994), 44-57.

14. See notes 6,7,8. Heschel, W. Lawson et al. "Abortion mortality, U.S., 1972-1987." *Am J Obstet Gynecol* (1994): 171:1365-72.

15. Cates, W., Jr. and Grimes, D. A. "Deaths from second trimester abortion by dilation and evacuation: causes, prevention, facilities." *J Am C Obstet Gynecol* (1981): 58:401.

16. Ney, Phillip G. "The relationship between abortion and child abuse." *Can J Psych* (1979): 24: 610-20.

17. Gullattee, A. C. "Psychiatric aspects of abortion." *J Nat Med Ass* (1973): 64:308-311.

18. *Catechism of the Catholic Church.* "Male and Female He Created Them," nn. 369-72.

19. National Federation for Catholic Youth Ministry. *True Love Waits.* Diocesan Resource Manual, p. 10.

20. Tufts Health Plan. Newsletter (November 1994).

21. Ursin, G. et al. "Oral contraceptive use and adenocarcinoma of the cervix." *The Lancet* (1994): 344: 1390-4.

22. Burke, Cormac. "Children and Values" in *Trust the Truth: A Symposium on the Twentieth Anniversary of the Encyclical Humanae Vitae* (Braintree, MA: Pope John XXIII Medical and Moral Center, 1991), 357-369.

23. Weissman, M.M. et al. "The epidemiology of depression; an update of sex differences in rates." *J Aff Dis* (1984): 7:179-88.

24. Pope John Paul II. Homily (Washington Mall, October 7, 1979).

25. *Catechism of the Catholic Church.* "The fecundity of marriage," n. 2370.

26. Ryder, R.E.J. "Natural Family Planning: effective birth control supported by the Catholic Church." *Brit Med J* (1993): 307.

27. Martin, Mary. "Infertility" in *Reproductive Endocrinology and Infertility* (Philadelphia, PA: J.P.Lippencott Co., 1994) vol. 5: 1025-36.

28. Neumann, Peter J. et al. "The cost of a successful delivery with In Vitro Fertilization." *NE J Med* (1994): 331:239-43.

29. Sherwin, Susan. *No Longer Patient: Feminist Ethics and Health Care* (Philadelphia, PA: Temple University Press, 1992), 135-6.

30. Grudzinskas, J. G. et al. "Commentary: Relocation of ectopic pregnancy to the uterine cavity: a dream or a reality?" *Brit J Obstet Gynecol* (1994): 101:651-2.

31. Stein, Margery. "Making babies or playing God?" *Family Circle* (September 20, 1994): 70.

32. Pope John Paul II. Address to Italian Medical Association (December 9, 1994). *L'Osservatore Romano*, English Edition (January 4, 1995): 8-9.

33. Pearce, J. M. et al. "Term delivery after intrauterine relocation of an ectopic pregnancy." *Brit J Obstet Gynecol* (1994): 101:716-7.

34. *Harvard Women's Health Watch* (November 1994): 1.

35. Angelo, E. Joanne. "Transforming a culture of death into a civilization of love." NCCB Respect Life Program (1993).

36. Pope John Paul II. Address to Health Care Leaders, Phoenix, Arizona. (September 14, 1987).

37. Pope John Paul II. *On the Christian Meaning Of Human Suffering* (February 11, 1984): no. 30.

38. Holtby, Winifred, quoted in Sommers, Christina H. *Who Stole Feminism? How Women Have Been Betrayed* (New York, NY: Simon and Schuster, 1994), 19.

39. Pope John Paul II. *Veritatis Spendor*. no. 118.

Chapter 10

PREACHING THE GOOD NEWS OF CATHOLIC MORALITY EFFECTIVELY

The Reverend Benedict J. Groeschel, C.F.R.

On the lintel of the church of St. Andrew across from the Federal Court House in Manhattan are inscribed the words, "Beati Qui Ambulant in Lege Domini." These words might well be a scriptural guide to the effective preaching of the moral teaching of the Catholic Church, especially as we are engaged in teaching the new *Catechism*. The negative corollary of this inscription is also a good guide, "Unblessed are they who do not walk according to the law of the Lord." A review of the history of Israel as well as an honest look at the history of the Church will reveal that when the people of God have been unfaithful en masse to the law of God and the moral demands of faith, catastrophe has resulted. As this century of holocausts and world wars draws to a close, the thoughtful observer might wonder why religious people so seldom see the relationship between moral relativism and global violence and disaster. A review of papal pronouncements in this century beginning with Pope Pius X on the eve of the First World War will reveal a strong and consistent attempt on the part of the popes to link together social ills and war on the one hand and moral relativism and hedonism on the other. There is observable an alarming pattern of the nations paying attention to Papal teachings too late and after the damage is done as is seen in Europe after the Second World War, when finally people who took the Church teaching seriously became heads of state.

The Obvious Signs of Decline

Nowhere is this moral insensitivity (shall we call it "blindness"?) more obvious at the moment than in the present Western industrialized nations, sometimes arrogantly referred to as the First World. The apostasy from faith linked with the so-called Enlightenment has spread far beyond the university and highly educated classes. The media has brought this apostasy into almost every nation and every home. For the first time in history the minds of children are formed not by the home, school and church, but by an elite band of entertainers, many of them morally dissolute and leading scandalous lives. These new folk heroes powerfully propagate values of selfism, sexual indulgence and violence. Many times this formula leads to self destruction through drugs, venereal disease or even suicide. And all the time the great fortunes and foundations of America and the wealthy European countries continue their relentless attack on family rights pushing one morally destructive agenda after another.

The result is not difficult to observe although its magnitude is lost on most of us, even on people in positions of pastoral responsibility in the various Western religious denominations. Just to give a brief statement of the present situation—among industrialized nations the

United States has the highest rate of crime and juvenile delinquency, the highest rate of unwanted pregnancy, the highest rate of venereal disease (45 million people with chronic incurable diseases, some of them fatal), a billion dollar pornography industry linked with the drug industry and along with all of this a stupendous addiction to drugs. Fifty percent of all marriages end in divorce. The Gay lobby exerts an influence vastly disproportionate to its actual membership which is estimated by all professional polls as less than two percent of the population. We have already mentioned the entertainment industry with its violence and actual encouragement of sexual irresponsibility and promiscuity. We could also mention the media's campaign against any influences by organized religion and especially against the Catholic Church and specifically against the clergy. A person would be foolish to think that this is a moment typical of the history of the United States. A few years ago when I was at the altar when St. Patrick's Cathedral was desecrated by a screaming mob during the middle of the Sunday pontifical mass, I realized that this was no longer business as usual.

The Enlightenment Leads to the Darkness

These societal problems do not come from nowhere. The Holy Father has consistently identified the source in the so-called Enlightenment with its rationalism, subjectivism, and its ultimate denial of the dignity of the individual, despite the fact that it began with what it conceived as an attempt to emancipate people from irrational social conventions. By propagating an ethic of total individual choice the Enlightenment two centuries ago undermined all sense of law and social responsibility and attempted to reduce Christianity merely to a medieval cultural survival. The Enlightenment did not mean to cause the present chaos, but as the Pope has pointed out in a number of places, the moral chaos of the twentieth century must be laid at its door. Indeed, the Holy Father bravely identifies the contemporary reruns of Enlightenment morality in his own country. Permit me to put in this quotation from *Crossing the Threshold of Hope*:

'God did not send His Son into the world to condemn the world but that the world might be saved through Him' (Jn 3:17). The world that the Son of Man found when He became man deserved condemnation, because of the sin that had dominated all of history, beginning with the fall of our first parents. This is another point that is absolutely unacceptable to post-enlightenment thought. It refuses to accept the reality of sin and in particular, it refuses to accept original sin. (p. 57)

The Holy Father encountered, interestingly enough, in his own country a good deal of resistance on this point. He continues:

When during my last visit to Poland, I chose the decalogue and the Commandment of Love as a theme for the homilies, all the Polish followers of the "enlightened agenda" were upset. For such people, the Pope becomes a persona non grata when he tries to convince the world of human sin. Objections of this sort conflict with much that St. John expresses in the words of Christ, who announced the coming of the Holy Spirit who will "convince the world in regard to sin" (Jn 16:8).

Parenthetically it is very worthwhile to mention that the whole notion of sin has been in decline in the Western industrialized nations for years. Thirty-five years ago the distinguished Protestant psychologist Carl Menninger asked this question in his book *Whatever Became of Sin*. Many times people have said to me in confession that they really can't think of any sins although they have been away from confession for years. Others say we thought there was no more original sin and that actual sin is difficult to commit. One professor of moral theology when asked to give an example of a venial sin said, "a single act of adultery." When this kind of thinking is disseminated among the faithful and even among seminarians, how can we expect that the Holy Spirit is going to be able to "convince the world in regard to sin"?

Selfism—The Predominant Ethic

The pervasive character of Enlightenment rationalism undermines the sense of transcendence on which religion is built. Soon afterwards followed moral relativism, then hedonism and selfism. It is worthwhile at this point to define selfism since it is the predominant social ethic in our country and its effects could be seen in the incredible thinking of the United States' presentations at the Cairo Conference on Population.

Selfism can be summarized as a social ethic with three simple but insidiously unchristian principles:

1. My first responsibility is to activate all my potentials for self-fulfillment and pleasure.

2. If the rights or needs of others (even my own children) stand in the way, I should put my own fulfillment first.

3. In some magical way the world owes it to me to give me all that I need to be completely fulfilled![1]

This ethic is both narcissistic and hedonistic recalling the philosophies that abounded in the declining Roman Empire. This ethic also contrasts sharply with the values of all reasonably successful civilizations of the last millennium (including the Christian West) where the ethic of the family predominated. Briefly stated, this ethic requires each generation to prepare the next so that life and human development can continue. It requires the children of the next generation to care for their parents and others of the preceding generation in old age and even by prayer to care for them in the next world. When the revelation of Christ, the Good News, was added to this ethic, there emerged easily what the Holy Father refers to as the ethic of love, an ethic in which a person only achieves complete fulfillment by complete self-donation. The Christian version of the universal family ethic is directly opposed to selfism.[2]

What Can the Church Do?

The task of the Church at present is to communicate the altruistic message of Christian morality based on the Agape of the Messiah to a culture saturated with selfism. It sounds like an impossible task and a great many of the clergy of all Christian denominations act like it is impossible. The faithful consistently complain that preaching and catechetical teaching is shallow, vague, lackluster, unrelated to the real challenges of life, unchallenging, and empty of that authority for which Our Lord Jesus Christ was known. If you doubt this ask one of your young relatives who has recently joined an evangelical church. No doubt the answer when you ask them will be, "I did not hear Christ preached in the Church." What is even more alarming is that it has been my experience after teaching in various seminaries for three decades that many seminarians and the handful of young religious sisters that one finds around are even more dissatisfied by the lack of a powerful evangelical challenge in their studies. They are deeply distressed with hearing endless lectures on what Jesus did not do, what Jesus did not say, what Jesus did not mean and what Jesus did not know. When those classes are over, they hear various things that in an unwarranted way minimize great teachings of the Church and disproportionally focus on other ones. Many are also fed a barrage of attacks against the teachings and person of the Holy Father. To a psychologist this endless negativism and program of constant religious deconstructionism are symptoms of the mass passive aggression that grips any social entity that is in deep conflict with itself. The question comes up immediately in one's mind: Did Christ come to make us comfortable or to show us the rough road to salvation?

Start With the Clergy and Teachers

A way must be found out of this malaise gripping so many preachers and teachers before they can even think of what to tell the faithful. It is my deep conviction after two decades of working with priests, deacons, religious and seminarians in therapy and spiritual direction that we must start with the clergy and with those in pastoral roles. They must be convinced of the reality of moral responsibility and of the necessity of a clear Christian rejection of selfism and hedonism. Then they will effectively preach to and teach the laity that the way to a genuine integrated fulfillment of one's individual humanity will come by a life of giving oneself in love according to the teachings of Christ as they are presented by those to whom Christ assigned to present these things, the successors of the Apostles.

Only after there is moral commitment by the teachers can we expect effective lessons to be given to the students. Goals define means. The goal is to have a society infiltrated by numbers of peoples committed to seeking fulfillment not by individualism or selfism but by a generous giving and following of the Gospel. There are two motives, one existential and the other eschatological, that we must keep in mind. I use the word existential here because the following of the Gospel brings peace and joy to the individual and the family even in the greatest of trials. We do not preach this fact. The devastating results of deliberately violating the divine law on character, personality and interpersonal relationships are not adequately recognized or enunciated. Of course a simple seriously repented fall rarely does much lasting harm. It can in fact be the cause of prayerful repentance and gratitude. Even a compulsive sin can give rise to a substantial conversion as one sees in the twelve step programs. But recognition of the evil, contrition and purpose of amendment are obviously necessary both theologically and psychologically.

Preaching and Teaching Reconciliation

For Catholics the sacrament of Reconciliation is an inestimable help in this struggle. But the use of this sacrament is in severe decline in the Western hemisphere and has almost disappeared in Catholic life in parts of northern Europe. When was the last time you heard a sermon on Confession? Our community makes Confession a center of our parish missions and I want to tell you, we catch some very big fish!

It is no use telling people about Confession when they are in middle age. They have to start when they are young and need someone to listen to them. I heard children's confessions all Saturday afternoon for 14 years at a children's treatment center and I never wasted one minute.

Disciples or Hired Hands?

Before we preach and teach in the name of Christ we must be His disciples. The disciple is very different from the churchman. The churchman or churchwoman asks, "what can I tell these people to keep them coming back?" The disciple asks, "how can I tell them what God wills me to tell them?" In His will is our peace fulfilled. This is the message of approximately one half of the parables of Christ: the sower, the ten virgins, the man with the vineyard. The other parables, the rich farmer, the story of Lazarus, and the Great Judgement in Matthew 25, all bring us to the eschatological side of preaching and teaching. I am convinced that before we can make any effective attempt at communicating the moral truths of the Christian faith we must make people aware of their eschatological responsibilities. These responsibilities are rooted in the very dignity of the human being as one called to eternal life who is free and responsible. May I read again from the book, *Crossing the Threshold of Hope*?

> Let us remember that not long ago, in sermons during retreats or missions, the Last Things—death, judgement, heaven, hell, or purgatory—were always a standard part of the program of meditation and preachers knew how to speak of them in an effective and evocative way. How many people were drawn to conversion and confession by these sermons and reflections on the Last Things! Furthermore, we have to recognize that this pastoral style was profoundly personal. 'Remember that at the end you will present yourself before God with your entire life. Before His judgement seat you will be responsible for all your actions, you will be judged not only on your actions and on your words but also on your thoughts, even the most secret.'
>
> It could be said that these sermons, which correspond perfectly to the content of Revelation in the Old and New Testaments, went to the very heart of man's inner world. They stirred his conscience, they threw him to his knees, they led him to the screen of the confessional, they had a profound saving effect all of their own. Man is free and therefore responsible. He has a personal and social responsibility, a responsibility before God, a responsibility which is his greatness. (p. 179)

153

True and False Teachers

Of course the ideas of a last judgement and of objective moral responsibility were completely anathema to the followers of the Enlightenment and still are. Several dogmas of the Catholic Faith which are defined are often subject to denial or very light treatment even by preachers, teachers and producers of religious textbooks. This unfortunately does an immense disservice to those who will, according to the words of Christ Himself, "have to render an account." I cannot imagine a worse injustice than not bringing to people's attention the fact that we must all stand before the judgement seat of God and experience what Christ describes so well in Matthew 25. The various immense social ills of our time ranging from the spread of global poverty to abortion and euthanasia all cry to heaven for justice, and justice will be done. It is not a matter of vengeance on the part of God but rather a reflection of His absolute truth and beauty. Fortunately we live in a time when the preaching of divine mercy is also extremely effective. But divine mercy must always be seen in conjunction with divine justice. One does not make sense without the other. And it is mercy that prevails ultimately but justice and righteousness are the foundations of the economy of salvation so well described in the new *Catechism.*

Where Do We Start—Four Steps

Where do we start? May I say very respectfully, we must start with bishops and especially diocesan bishops who are responsible for the care of souls more than anyone else. This is a difficult and daunting task. My impression is that the first step is to preach to the clergy and make it eminently clear that every priest and pastoral person in the diocese is responsible to teach the teachings of the Church and to live them. If they are lived, they will be preached and if they are not lived the faithful will see through the hypocrisy of false teaching. Secondly, a very serious look must be had at religious education at all levels. This must begin with textbooks and go right through to the materials made available under diocesan auspices for the continuing education of the clergy. We sin both by commission and omission. If a vibrant and convincing presentation of the new *Catechism* is lacking, I do not see how a pastor could hold himself exempt from a serious responsibility for negligence.

Thirdly, the laity must hear from the pulpit and in instructions that the way to a happy and blessed life is clearly revealed in Scripture to be the following of the law of the Lord. Pastorally responsible people must follow the law themselves. They cannot indulge in the debauched entertainment provided by the media and hope to have a clear conscience. They cannot indulge themselves in affluence while more and more people in our society are born below the level of poverty. They cannot hold themselves exempt from a responsibility to speak out on burning moral and social issues of our time beginning with the right to life. Often I hear priests say, "Well, I don't agree with this way of protesting and I don't agree with that." Fine, but what do they agree to do and are they doing it?

Fourthly, it is an eminently clear fact in the Gospel that no one can be a disciple of Christ without prayer and interiority. Superficiality is as much a contradiction of the Gospel as injustice is. The living of the moral and theological virtues and especially such sensitive virtues as chastity, modesty, diligence and generosity, is not easy in our hedonistic culture. It requires us frankly to be countercultural. We cannot expect to be understood or applauded. It is quite obvious that those who live up to these virtues are secretly admired, even by the children of this world. Witness the popularity of Mother Teresa.

Fields White for the Harvest

My preaching takes me around the country and even to some of the other countries represented at this meeting. Everywhere I go I find very devout lay people who have maintained a loyal discipleship to the Gospel often in the face of clerical scandal and pastoral negligence. I find many enthusiastic young people, most of them converts from a dissolute way of life who are anxious to follow the Gospel with fervor and enthusiasm. It is amazing the number of young couples that one meets who embrace the Church's teaching on contraception and see it as something that makes their marriage more meaningful and all the more sacred. There are many others, even a larger number, who stand on the side with wide eyes. They are looking to see. Do we believe what we say? Are we willing to try to practice it? Are we willing to show to others that adherence to the Gospel and the teaching of the Church is a road that leads to blessedness in this life and to eternal beatitude in the next. They are watching. Why do we pay so much attention to the minority of dissolute minstrels who run the media? There are a large numbers of people deeply dissatisfied with great loneliness and alienation caused by selfishness in our society who hope for something that is meaningful. This explains the immense popularity of Pope John Paul II in spite of the religious decline of our time and the ceaseless attacks on the teaching authority of the church and the pastoral office of the successor of St. Peter.

Bishops, may I respectfully remind each one of you as I remind myself that in a few years of this earth's time each one of us will stand before the judgement seat of God. We must render an account of our works. Whatever office or dignities we have in this life will be put into the scale. They will be seen not as credits but debits, blessings for which we must give an account because from those to whom much is given much will be expected.

I am very grateful and honored by this opportunity to address the successors of the Apostles. With utmost loyalty to the Church and respect for the office of bishop I submit these recommendations. They are comprehensive but I hope realistic. I think there is a way out of the present morass but it depends on the free will of every believing Christian and especially every believing priest and bishop. In a recent study in the *New York Times* the Catholic Church was described as a church at risk. Branches of the Catholic Church at risk in the past have perished as they did in northern Europe. In other countries they rallied themselves. One of the most intense pieties in the world existed in northern Italy just below the Alps where the Church had to marshal its forces as the ideas of the Reformation swept down over the Alps. This very fertile field of Catholicism in northern Italy has provided the majority of the great Popes of modern times. We ourselves could, out of the moral chaos of our times, bring a vibrant and admirable Catholicism. Do not be disheartened with the fact that we are dealing with a dysfunctional population filled with dysfunctional families. It was to the nameless, faceless, rootless populations of the pagan Roman empire that the Church preached the Gospel with great effectiveness at the time of the decline of the empire. Perhaps we live in times that are somewhat analogous. My own experience is that out in that nameless, faceless, rootless crowd are people who have been severely deprived of love, of faith, and of hope but who thirst for these virtues. There are many earnest and hungry souls whom God will call despite their scars to embrace the salvation that comes from the Gospel and from belief and trust in Jesus Christ.

Notes

1. See D. Yankelovich, *New Rules* (New York: Random House, 1981), p. 6, for an excellent analysis of Selfism.

2. I see the collapse of many religious communities in Western civilization as a very good example of the effects of selfism on a naïve Christian environment. The root cause for the decline of religious life was an acceptance of the ethic of selfism without qualification. How often in some communities does one see great self-giving on the part of one religious in complete conflict with the selfism of the next. It's a rerun of the old adage that "the corruption of the best is the worst." Of course there are a great many religious in the middle of this, deeply conflicted and now filled with resentment over that conflict. (See my book, *Reform of Renewal* [Ignatius Press, 1990].)

Chapter 11

THE *ETHICAL AND RELIGIOUS DIRECTIVES FOR CATHOLIC HEALTH CARE SERVICES:* A COMMENTARY

Peter J. Cataldo, Ph.D.

Continuing a tradition which had its beginnings in 1921 with the code of ethics for the Catholic Hospital Association of the United States, Catholic health care once again has a set of ethical and religious directives revised in response to the changing needs of this ministry. I will refer to these *Ethical and Religious Directives for Catholic*

Health Care Services as the *Directives*. A brief commentary on this set of seventy Directives with an Appendix must necessarily be selective. As for general comment, I may say that having been a part of the Pope John Center's consultation on the *Directives* since the first draft, I have observed the progression from a document which was primarily an educational document in the beginning to a final document of directives within an educational framework. The latter sort of document is that which will best serve the Catholic health care ministry. Quite appropriately the document provides a set of directives for action, and at the same time provides needed and helpful explanations about the Catholic teaching underlying the individual Directives. Most of the Directives are able to stand alone on their own merits, which I believe is preferable for a document of this sort. But in the case of some Directives there is an internal dependency upon other Directives which might possibly prove inconvenient as we shall see.

The goal of my presentation is to give brief commentaries on specific topics in the *Directives* that have traditionally received particular attention within the Catholic health care community by clarifying their meaning in some cases, and by pointing out potential difficulties in others. My commentaries are not intended as suggestions for revision, but rather as suggestions for ways of interpretation. This sort of presentation requires a close examination of the text. I will not be taking the approach of Roper in Robert Bolt's *A Man for All Seasons* when he says in response to More's query about the King's oath: "We don't need to know the wording—we know what it will mean!"[1]

I
Science, Technology, and Catholic Moral Teaching

It is often stated in bioethics that the development of medical science and technology in the 20th century and certainly in the second half of this century has challenged and raced ahead of the moral tradition in health care, that this tradition is ill-equipped to resolve the remarkable and rapid advances in biotechnology. It is widely thought that traditional moral obligations in medicine such as the obligations to conserve human life and to do no harm, and principles like the principle of the double effect can no longer provide the guidance they once did in the face of technologies which enable medicine to prolong human life longer than was ever previously expected. In fact many health care professionals and bioethicists consider compliance with these obligations and principles in certain types of cases to be detrimental to the practice of good medicine.

If the Church is to promulgate a set of Directives for the ethical and religious standards in Catholic health care, it must address at the outset the common assumption that traditional ethics in medicine is superannuated. It must show that the moral teaching and tradition of the Church is not in principle anti-science and anti-technology. The *Directives* do precisely this in the General Introduction where it states:

> The dialogue between medical science and Christian faith has for its primary purpose the common good of all human persons. It presupposes that science and faith do not contradict each other. Both are grounded in respect for truth and freedom. As new knowledge and new technologies expand, each person must form a correct conscience based on the moral norms for proper health care.[2]

The Church's understanding of the nature of human activity is the key to her view of the balance between the moral criteria for science and technology on the one hand, and their methodology on the other. This is so because science and technology originate from, and are directed toward, human activity. In this way the Church recognizes that science and technology are at the service of human nature and the activity which fulfills that nature. *Gaudium et Spes* explains that:

> Human activity proceeds from man: it is also ordered to him. When he works, not only does he transform matter and society, but he fulfills himself. He learns, he develops his faculties, and he emerges from and transcends himself.... Technological progress may supply the material for human advance but it is powerless to actualize it.

> Here then is the norm for human activity—to harmonize with the authentic interests of the human race, in accordance with God's will and design, and to enable men as individuals and as members of society to pursue and fulfil their total vocation. (no. 35)[3]

Given the intrinsic requirements of science and technology for moral direction, and in particular, given the relation between technological progress and human activity, it is important to make clear to the users of the *Directives* that there is nothing unreasonable or unwarranted about the Church's aim to provide ethical and religious directives.

Social Justice and Catholic Health Care

The final version of the *Directives* also achieved a balance between the social responsibility of Catholic health care and the moral teachings of the Church. Given the tension between the sometimes fierce competition for patient populations and the need to serve the poor, there emerges a real temptation to reduce the identity of Catholic health care to social justice. The enumeration of the normative principles of social responsibility and the corresponding Directives, found in Part I and entitled "The Social Responsibility of Catholic Health Care Services," include a call for adherence to the moral teachings of the Church in the midst of meeting the social responsibilities of Catholic health care. The "right to the means for the proper development of life such as adequate health care," the provision of "adequate health care for the poor," the contribution of Catholic health care to the common good, and the "responsible stewardship of health care resources," cannot be achieved in a manner contrary to the moral teaching of the Church according to the principles and Directives of Part I. This balance reflects previous statements of the NCCB, in particular the documents *Health and Health Care* (1981) and the *Resolution on Health Care Reform* (1993). The identity of Catholic health care is neither reduced to social morality nor to individual morality in those documents. For example, in the *Resolution on Health Care Reform*, the bishops acknowledge that "[w]e are deeply concerned that Catholic and other institutions with strong moral foundations may face increasing economic and regulatory pressures to compromise their moral principles and to participate in practices inconsistent with their commitment to human life."[4] In response to the social context of Catholic health care, Directive 6 explicitly recognizes the ordering of social and moral elements within the

161

common good: "[c]ollaboration with other health care providers, in ways that do not compromise Catholic social and moral teaching, can be an effective means of...stewardship."

With respect to the problem of reducing Catholic identity to social justice, it is important to recognize that the notion of the common good is comprised of two reciprocally related parts: the social good and the individual good. The common good is not achieved to the extent that either of its component parts go unfulfilled. Jacques Maritain explained well the reciprocity of individual and social morality in the concept of the common good. He wrote about the common good that:

> It is the good human life of the multitude, of a multitude of persons; it is their communion in good living...it presupposes the persons and flows back upon them, and, in this sense, is achieved in them...it includes the sum or sociological integration of all the civic conscience, political virtues and sense of right and liberty, of all the activity, material property and spiritual riches, of unconsciously operative hereditary wisdom, of moral rectitude, justice, friendship, happiness, virtue and heroism in the individual lives of its members.[5]

Echoing *Gaudium et Spes*, the *Catechism of the Catholic Church* states that "[f]irst, the common good presupposes respect for the person as such...Society should permit each of its members to fulfill his vocation" (no. 1907). *Gaudium et Spes* itself states that "The social order and its development must constantly yield to the good of the person, since the order of things must be subordinate to the order of persons and not the other way around..." (no. 26). Given that the common good flows back upon the totality of the person in his or her human vocation, any actions of health care providers which are contrary to the personal moral goods of the individual, such as the goods of the transmission of human life, cannot validly be made in the name of the common good.

Conscience and the Directives

Part Three of the *Directives* stresses the importance of conscience in the relationship between the health care professional and the patient. As a balance was achieved in Part I on the "Social Responsibility of Catholic Health Care Services," so too the ninth and final draft the Directives achieved a balance between, on the one hand, respect for the conscience of the health care provider, and, on the other, respect for the conscience of the patient. The interpersonal relationship between professional and patient is centered on a recognition of the patient's conscience and convictions about his own health care and the professional's moral responsibilities, including his or her responsibility to the Catholic identity of the institution in which he works. The Introduction to Part Three explains the unique personal contribution that the professional and patient each make to their relationship:

> The health care professional has the knowledge and experience to pursue the goals of healing, the maintenance of health, and the compassionate care of the dying, taking into account the patient's convictions and spiritual needs, and the moral responsibilities of all concerned.... The patient, in turn, has a responsibility to use these physical and mental resources in the service of moral and spiritual goals to the best of his or her ability.[6]

As this text indicates, the interpersonal, professional-patient relationship is also constituted by an objective element. The person whom Catholic health care serves has a readily identifiable dignity the whole of which, not merely one or another part, must be respected. This objective dimension to the relationship between professional and patient is captured in the remainder of the Introduction to Part III:

> When the health care professional and the patient use institutional Catholic health care, they also accept its public commitment to the church's understanding of and witness to the dignity of the human person. The church's moral teaching on health care nurtures a truly interpersonal professional-patient relationship. This professional-patient relationship is never separated, then, from the Catholic identity of the health care institution. The faith that inspires Catholic health care guides

medical decisions in ways that fully respect the dignity of the person and the relationship with the health care professional.[7]

Not only do the Directives concerning the professional-patient relationship reflect the subjective and objective components of the relationship, but they also show that there is a moral ordering of the former to the latter. Directives 24, 25, and 28 show that the patient's wishes are to be followed in both honoring advance medical directives and in a patient's decisions in conscience about treatment up to the point of conflict with Catholic moral teaching:

> ...The institution, however, will not honor an advance directive that is contrary to Catholic teaching. (no. 24)

> ...Decisions by the designated surrogate should be faithful to Catholic moral principles and to the person's intentions and values, or if the person's intentions are unknown, to the person's best interests. (no. 25)

> ...The free and informed health care decision of the person or the person's surrogate is to be followed so long as it does not contradict Catholic principles. (no. 28)

It is helpful to understand that the dual components of the professional-patient relationship are parallel to the subjective and objective components of conscience itself, upon which the relationship is built. Contrary to the popular notion that conscience is an absolutely autonomous capacity to sanction whatever moral feelings one may experience, conscience is an act which is open to the very ground of man's being, to paraphrase Joseph Cardinal Ratzinger at this Workshop.[8] The pursuit of what is good on the part of professional and patient can only arise from who they are as human beings. "From its origin," Cardinal Ratzinger writes, "man's being resonates with some things and clashes with others."[9] Conscience is like a primordial memory, an anamnesis of the origin of our being in God the infinite Good. "This anamnesis of the origin," he explains further, "which results from the godlike constitution of our being is not a conceptually articulated knowing, a store of retrievable contents. It is so to speak an inner sense, a capacity to recall...."[10] The *Catechism of the Catholic Church* similarly describes conscience as a "...witness to the authority of truth in reference to the supreme Good to which the

164

human person is drawn, and it welcomes the commandments. When he listens to his conscience, the prudent man can hear God speaking" (no. 1777). By its witness to the whole of human dignity, the identity of Catholic health care serves both to provide the objective content of the moral dimension of the professional-patient relationship, and serves as an instructive and formative influence on the consciences of professionals and patients. Understood from this perspective the *Directives* have a critical function in the relationship between Catholic health care's mission and conscience.

The Inseparable Meanings of the Conjugal Act and Reproductive Technologies

The Introduction to Part IV of the *Directives*, "Issues in Care for the Beginning of Life," gives testimony to the profound and rich teaching of the Church on the place of conjugal love within marriage. Among its many quotations from magisterial documents on the nature and morality of conjugal love, the Introduction quotes the teaching of Paul VI in *Humanae Vitae* on the inseparability of the unitive and procreative meanings of the conjugal act. Paragraph 12 of *Humanae Vitae* states that:

> The doctrine that the Magisterium of the Church has often explained is this: there is an unbreakable connection [*nexu indissolubili*] between the unitive meaning and the procreative meaning [of the conjugal act], and both are inherent in the conjugal act. This connection was established by God, and Man is not permitted to break it through his own volition.[11]

All of the Directives on the use of reproductive technologies except Directive 39 are based upon the inseparability of the unitive and procreative meanings of the conjugal act. Directive 39 states the conditions under which techniques for infertility therapy would be permissible. The first condition is that the techniques "...respect the unitive and procreative meanings of sexual intercourse" (no. 39). However, the wording of this condition in Directive 39 is inconsistent with the Introduction and with Directives 38 and 41, in so far as it does not make explicit reference to the inseparability of the twofold meaning of the conjugal act.

Emphasis on the inseparability element is particularly important for an ethical evaluation of reproductive technologies. Most well-intentioned couples seeking to use reproductive technology have experienced a long agonizing trial of waiting to conceive. The spouses love each other and love children. They have a sincere desire to have a family of their own. They believe that having a child through *in vitro* fertilization or some other similar reproductive technology achieves the good of bringing new life into the world and the good of transforming their love to the level of parenthood. Moreover, they believe either implicitly or explicitly that their marriage gives them a right to a child. All of these factors are the ingredients for couples to claim or assume that their use of prohibited reproductive technologies is fulfilling the unitive and procreative meanings of marital love.

But the love which produces a child by means of a prohibited procedure is neither unitive nor procreative. The separation of these two elements corrupts each. It is not unitive because the child which results from their actions is not the fruit of a complete self-giving in which each spouse has given all that each is for the other in a conjugal act. Even though a child is brought to life, their actions are not procreative. A child has been "reproduced" but not procreated in cooperation with the "holy laws of God" for the transmission of human life. Precisely because the spouses do not act in communion with each other according to the inherent nature of spousal love, their actions are not truly said to be procreative.

I believe that the turning point for many couples considering the use of *in vitro* procedures comes with the realization that their marriage does not give them a right to a child, that to take such a stance is, in the words of *Donum vitae*, to consider the child "as an object of ownership" rather than as "a gift, 'the supreme gift' and the most gratuitous gift of marriage, and…a living testimony of the mutual giving of his parents" (II, B, 8). This realization is at the same time a recognition that the child's human dignity demands that he or she be conceived by a conjugal act whose unitive and procreative aspects are inseparable. To understand that the child is not an object of domination is to understand that "the generation of a child," as explained by *Donum Vitae*, "must therefore be the fruit of that mutual giving which is realized in the conjugal act wherein the spouses cooperate as servants and not as masters in the work of the Creator who is Love" (II, B, 4).

The Early Induction of Labor

There are two Directives which pertain to the early induction of maternal labor. They are Directive 47, which indirectly refers to early induction, and Directive 49:

> 47. Operations, treatments and medications that have as their direct purpose the cure of a proportionately serious pathological condition of a pregnant woman are permitted when they cannot be safely postponed until the unborn child is viable, even if they will result in the death of the unborn child.[12]

> 49. For a proportionate reason, labor may be induced after the fetus is viable.

Although the two Directives refer respectively to inducing labor (among other things) before viability and after viability, they are grounded in the same moral principles and are applied with prudential judgment in cases according to those same principles. Those principles are the inviolability of human life and the obligation to conserve the lives of mother and child to the extent possible under the circumstances. According to these principles in the case of a child with anomalies incompatible with life *ex utero*, the child's life ought to be maintained *in utero* so long as the pregnancy is not causing harm either to the child or to the mother. This can be the case, for example, with anencephalic fetuses.[13]

However, some argue that any emotional trauma or anguish on the part of the mother in these cases qualifies as a proportionate reason to induce labor either before or after viability. This is where a specification about the type of reason considered proportionate, or at least a qualification about what is not considered proportionate, would have been helpful. For, to argue that emotional anguish which is not causing physical harm to mother or child is a proportionate reason, is to assume that a child can be treated as an object of another's pleasure or displeasure. Inducing labor in this case is an act of hastening death as a means toward the purpose of ending the grief. But the inherent, absolute dignity of the child cannot be made relative by the circumstances of the case, traumatic as they may be. Moreover, footnote 32 at the end of Directive 49 does not appear helpful in resolving this problem since *Donum Vitae* I, 2, to which the note refers, is on prenatal diagnosis and makes no mention of maternal labor or its early induction.[14]

Sacrificing Functional Integrity

Directive 29 on the permissibility of sacrificing the functional integrity of the body is critically important not only for providing the moral justification of medical and surgical treatment, but also for its implications about stewardship of the body in general and its implications for treatments which induce sterility. The Directive states that:

> 29. All persons served by Catholic health care have the right and duty to protect and preserve their bodily and functional integrity. The functional integrity of the person may be sacrificed to maintain the health or life of the person when no other morally permissible means is available.

It will be helpful to look at the philosophical foundation of the Directive in the thought of St.Thomas Aquinas. He explained the relations of the parts of the body to the whole, according to what is now called the principle of totality, in this way:

> Since a member is a part of the whole human body, it is for the sake of the whole, as the imperfect is for the sake of the perfect. Hence a member of the human body is to be disposed of according as it is expedient for the whole body. Now a member of the human body is of itself [*per se*] useful to the good of the whole body, yet accidentally [*per accidens*] it may happen to be hurtful, as when a decayed member is a source of corruption to the whole body.[15]

The human body exists as a whole, as a subsisting unity, and as such is the end and final cause of its constituent parts. The existence and function of the individual parts are fully intelligible only in relation to the whole of the body as their end and fulfillment. This means that the parts of the body act primarily and directly for the good of the whole and for themselves only in a secondary way. Even those elements which are capable of existing apart from the body do not exist precisely as substances unto themselves but exist in altered states according to their subordination to the whole. Aquinas' principle that the imperfect is for the sake of the perfect still holds for a modern advancement like tissue culture and banking. Although human tissue can be maintained outside of the body, only part of its potential is utilized by virtue of the absence of a whole body to which it would otherwise contribute its function, and thus is correctly said to be in an imperfect state. Since the various parts of the body exist in a subordinated relation to the whole, they may be affected by medical and surgical treatment, depending on the circumstances, so as to serve better the good of the whole.

The finality which characterizes the relation of the parts of the body to the whole, also points up the difference between stewardship and dominion over the body. The inherent finality of function is something independent of the will and thus demands a stance of stewardship, not one of domination. Pope Pius XII explained well the connection of stewardship to totality in his allocution to the First International Congress of Histopathology:

> As far as the patient is concerned, he is not absolute master of himself, of his body, or of his soul. He cannot, therefore, freely dispose of himself as he pleases. Even the motive for which he acts is not by itself either sufficient or determining. The patient is bound by the immanent purposes fixed by nature. He possesses the right to use, limited by natural finality, the faculties and powers of his human nature. Because he is the beneficiary, and not the proprietor, he does not possess unlimited power to allow acts of destruction or of mutilation of anatomic or functional character.[16]

Pius XII goes on to conclude that by virtue of the principle of totality, an individual may give parts of the body to destruction or mutilation to assure existence, to avoid serious problems, and to treat them.

The final version of Directive 29 also has a very important footnote, number 17, which refers the reader to Directive 53 on direct and indirect sterilization. I believe that without this footnote the wording of Directive 29 could be easily interpreted to allow for the sacrificing of the functional integrity of the reproductive organs to maintain physical or psycho-social health which might be jeopardized by a future pregnancy. Use of the term "morally permissible" to qualify the means employed to maintain health and life was not by itself sufficient in the previous versions to preclude misinterpretation. In fact, it could be argued that the expression "other morally permissible means" assumes that this sacrifice is moral by virtue of the presumption that there are no morally permissible means other than the sacrifice. While the intent of the sentence is correct, its structure inadequately expresses that intent by not making it evident *why* this particular type of sacrifice is morally acceptable, as is assumed. The addition of footnote 17 in the final version provides the criteria for what Directive 29 allows. However, a case still might be made that the text of the Directive should itself express the criteria. In any event, showing the relevance of footnote 17 for Directive 29 will be an important part of educating the users of the *Directives.*

The Duty to Preserve Life

Part V of the *Directives* on "Issues in Care for the Dying" gives witness to the Christian meaning of suffering and death and outlines the essential moral principles of Catholic teaching on care for the dying and on judgments about life-sustaining treatment. There are two points about Part V that warrant some attention. The first concerns the explanation of the moral obligation to preserve life. The Introduction to Part V states:

> ...We have a duty to preserve our life, and to use it for the glory of God; but the duty to preserve life is not absolute, for we may reject life-prolonging procedures that are insufficiently beneficial or excessively burdensome. Suicide and euthanasia are never morally acceptable options.

> The task of medicine is to care even when it cannot cure.[17]

It is true that, in the words of the Introduction, we "do not have absolute power over life" for only God has such power. But it is not true that because "we may reject life-prolonging procedures that are insufficiently beneficial or excessively burdensome," there is no absolute duty to preserve life. The absence of an absolute duty does not follow from the fact that it is morally licit to refuse treatment.

That there is an absolute duty to preserve life and what that means is evident from the *Directives* themselves and from Church teaching on this matter. The absolute moral norm against taking innocent human life and the duty to preserve life are correlative principles. If there is not an absolute moral duty to preserve human life, then how do we justify the proscriptions against euthanasia, suicide, and assisted-suicide, and the prescriptions for effective pain management, proportionate means of preserving life, and continued care for the dying ? In the absence of an absolute duty to preserve human life the obligation never to take life directly is incomplete. Innocent human life must never be directly taken because it must be cared for and preserved or conserved in due measure to the circumstances. If the duty to preserve life were not itself absolute, then the duty never to take innocent human life would be untenable since the reason for the prohibition would no longer exist. The two sets of obligations are the positive and negative sides of what is due to the human being.[18] The *Declaration on Euthanasia* after explaining the conditions under which it is morally permissible to forgo or withdraw treatment adds the following condition: "so long as the normal care due to the sick person in similar cases is not interrupted" (IV). The normal care referred to is the concrete fulfillment of the obligation to preserve life under the circumstances of the life being cared for as described in the document.[19]

We may "reject life-prolonging procedures that are insufficiently beneficial or excessively burdensome" for the reason that they are a means of preserving life disproportionate to the condition of the life being preserved, not because the duty to preserve human life is not absolute. It is the *disproportion* which we reject, not the effort to preserve life. We are under the very same obligation to preserve human life in the case of the dying patient as we are for a healthy person; the difference lies in the means we should use to fulfill that obligation. The obligation as such remains absolute; the means of fulfilling that duty are relative to the circumstances of the life being preserved.

The actions of giving nursing care, comfort care, and effective analgesics after forgoing or withdrawing more aggressive forms of care are all positive measures and forms of preserving or conserving human life in fulfillment of the obligation. These measures are undertaken precisely because the obligation is still in force. Part of the problem of recognizing the absolute character of the obligation is perhaps due to the word "preserve." St. Thomas Aquinas uses *conservere*, to explain this positive precept of the natural law, which can be translated as "preserve" or "conserve."[20] It would seem preferable to use the word "conserve." The use of "conserve" in English perhaps has a more flexible connotation than "preserve" corresponding to the concrete fulfillment of the obligation. It is also helpful to remember that the negative precepts of the natural law are fulfilled in only one way, i.e., by not performing the prohibited act. Positive precepts are fulfilled in any number of ways, but this fact does not take away the absolute binding character of some precepts such as the duty to conserve life.[21]

Another reason for the absolute nature of the obligation to conserve human life is that in the present culture of death, with its strong forces pushing for euthanasia and physician-assisted suicide, a clear and contrasting defense of the Church's moral teaching on end-of-life issues must be made. Many Catholics and non-Catholics are confused about the meaning of the Church's teaching and find no real difference in the common distinction between "killing and allowing to die" which is made on behalf of that teaching. I submit that the distinction itself is a false one and does not serve well as a justification of the Church's teaching. The distinction is a false one because "allowing to die" is a negative, secondary effect of some other positive action and is not the proper concept to make in contradistinction with "killing" which directly refers to a positive action. An opposite positive action needs to be contrasted with killing in order to show the true difference between euthanasia and Catholic teaching on the question. The distinction is better understood within the context of the acting agents and what they do, and not simply from the perspective of the effects of their actions. Thus the Church's teaching on care for the dying is properly characterized by the distinction between killing and conserving human life by proportionate means.

A second area of clarification might be needed with respect to Directives 56, 57, and 59. Directives 56 and 57 are as follows:

56. A person has a moral obligation to use ordinary or proportionate means of preserving his or her life. Proportionate means are those that in the judgment of the patient offer a reasonable hope of benefit and do not entail an excessive burden, or impose excessive expense on the family or the community.

57. A person may forgo extraordinary or disproportionate means of preserving life. Disproportionate means are those that in the patient's judgment do not offer a reasonable hope of benefit or entail an excessive burden, or impose excessive expense on the family, or the community.

Directives 56 and 57 respectively are intended to provide universal definitions of ethically ordinary and extraordinary means of conserving life. A potential problem arises not with the separate elements of these definitions but with an internal inconsistency between the objective and subjective aspects of the definitions arising from their wording. The Directives attempt to provide an objective standard of reasonableness with respect to what is and is not a hope of benefit and an excessive burden. Yet at the same time the wording of the definitions could be interpreted as a reduction of the objective elements of the standard to the subjective judgement of the patient.

Any use of an objective standard of reasonableness is vitiated by the fact that what is reasonable is explicitly said to be what the patient judges to be reasonable. Unlike what is found in Part IV of the *Declaration on Euthanasia*, to which Directives 56 and 57 make reference, these Directives could be read as confusing the distinction between an objective standard of reasonableness and the subjective application or judgement of that standard in a particular case. The patient judges what is reasonable, not in the sense of creating a standard of reasonableness for himself or herself, as can be interpreted by the wording of the Directives, but rather in the sense of judging how certain objective criteria of health relate to the particular circumstances of the patient's condition.

Directive 59 on the other hand does recognize the distinction. It reads as follows:

> The free and informed judgment made by a competent adult patient concerning the use or withdrawal of life-sustaining procedures should always be respected and normally complied with, unless it is contrary to Catholic moral teaching.

The inclusion of a condition prohibiting compliance with a patient's judgement in this Directive is a recognition of the fact that the objective criteria of what is reasonable is not made by an absolute determination of the patient. A benign reading of these three Directives would find that Directive 59 completes 56 and 57. But if the Directives are meant to stand on their own merits, as seems to be the case, Directives 56 and 57 are inconsistent with Directive 59 on the role of the subjective judgment of the patient.

The Appendix of the *Directives*

The Appendix, which is titled "The Principles Governing Cooperation," is a potentially valuable addition to the *Directives*.[22] In particular, the recognition of "implicit formal cooperation" is, in my opinion, critically important. The complexity of the corporate relationships in the new partnerships make the Catholic health care providers vulnerable to a formal cooperation with wrongdoing which is implicit or indirect. No longer is it necessary to establish formal cooperation only on the basis of a direct approval of the wrongdoing of another. The Appendix of the *Directives* shows that the new partnerships have generated a new model of formal cooperation. These formal relationships have opened the possibility of Catholic providers giving approval to prohibited procedures by helping to create the very formal conditions which make the procedures possible. By participating in the formulation of, and by assenting to, any by-laws or formal agreements which establish the corporate structures that provide for the prohibited procedures, the Catholic provider has created the very conditions which give reality to the causes of the wrong actions. It is in and through these relationships that the implicit character of the formal cooperation is present.

In light of these considerations the use of the term "object" in the explanation of implicit formal cooperation might not be specific enough for a proper understanding of this concept. To the non-theologian the language of "object" might very well refer to the subjective intention of the parties involved. The "object" of the cooperator might be interpreted to mean, for instance, the subjective intent to continue health care to the poor which would be understood as not intending the "object" of the wrongdoer. However, there might still be a formal cooperation in so far as the Catholic provider has participated in the formal conditions which make possible the wrong actions. It is by understanding the issue on the level of the formal conditions of the prohibited actions that the explanation of implicit formal cooperation in terms of the cooperator's and the wrongdoer's "objects" can be rightly interpreted; but this is not immediately apparent from the wording of the Appendix.

A final observation about the use of the term "distant" in the Appendix to explain material cooperation should also be made. Use of the term "distant" in the context of cooperation with prohibited procedures that occur at some particular location leaves its meaning open to a quantitative interpretation. I have already alluded to the fact that even though measures are taken to have prohibited procedures performed somewhere geographically "distant" from the Catholic provider, formal cooperation can still occur. In order to avert such an interpretation, I would suggest explaining the use of "distant" as meaning that the material cooperation should be as "causally removed" as possible from the wrongdoer's act. Understanding "distant" to mean "causally removed" bases the moral evaluation of cooperation on the causes of the act, which is where moral responsibility lies.

II

Implementing the *Directives* in a Pluralistic World

At several points the prescriptive force of the *Directives* is clearly indicated. The Preamble states that one of the two purposes of the Directives is "to provide authoritative guidance on certain moral issues which face Catholic health care today." The second section of each of the six parts is described in the Preamble as being in "prescriptive form." The General Introduction refers to the Church providing "normative guidance and direction" on many moral questions. Directives 5 and 9 directly and explicitly declare the obligatory force of the *Directives*:

> 5. Catholic health care services must adopt these directives as policy, require adherence to them within the institution as a condition for medical privileges and employment, and provide appropriate instruction regarding the directives for administration, medical and nursing staff and other personnel.

> 9. Employees of a Catholic health care institution must respect and uphold the religious mission of the institution and adhere to these directives. They should maintain professional standards and promote the institution's commitment to human dignity and the common good.

One of the problems which educational efforts on the *Directives* will immediately face is the objection that a document of directives cannot legitimately be enforced in a pluralistic society. The fifth normative principle articulated in the Introduction to Part I provides an important foundation from which to respond to the expected objection:

> Fifth, within a pluralistic society, Catholic health care services will encounter requests for medical procedures contrary to the moral teachings of the church. Catholic health care does not offend the rights of individual conscience by refusing to provide or permit medical procedures that are judged morally wrong by the teaching authority of the church.[23]

There are two points to be made about the pluralism objection. First, an acceptance of the political and sociological facts that society consists of a wide diversity of cultural, ethnic, and religious systems and beliefs need not be an acceptance of moral relativism as well. This is a confusion which is commonly made and it is no different for those working in health care. The plurality of society does not equate to a plurality in the nature of truth itself and moral truth in particular. What the pluralism objection really states is that the enforcement of a set of Catholic health care directives is illegitimate because the presumption of an objective order of moral truth by the *Directives* is illegitimate. But Catholic health care cannot fairly be criticized for holding a presupposition which its critics merely assume to be false. The pluralism objection looks something like this: 1) society at large and the health care world in particular are pluralistic; 1a) suppressed premise: socio-political pluralism is equivalent to moral relativism; 2) the Catholic health care directives are in conflict with a plurality of views; 3) therefore, the directives cannot be accepted. In effect the argument is stating that the Catholic directives cannot be accepted because they are not morally relativistic; but moral relativism is precisely a position which the Church need not accept.

Another point to be made about the pluralism issue is that it is sometimes claimed that because Catholic health care operates within a pluralistic society, its adherence to ethical and religious directives constitutes "bad medicine" in many cases. This argument also assumes that so-called good medicine is ethically neutral. A desired procedure, though it be prohibited by the *Directives*, is considered an ethically neutral matter and therefore any prohibition of it is a deprivation of something to which the patient is reasonably entitled. In reality this is a conflict between two different views of what is considered ethical medicine. The fact that the opposing view finds acceptable whatever is considered unacceptable by the Catholic hospital, means that it is advancing an ethical view different from that of the hospital's— not that the opposing view is ethically neutral while the hospital's is not. What the opposing view would allow is done so ultimately because the procedure is considered more suitable to and compatible with the patient as a human person than what the hospital believes is for the good of the patient. As a conflict of two differing moral views of medicine, the *Directives* are correct to state that there is no offence against the rights of conscience when Catholic health care exercises its conscience. An important first step toward resolving this facet of the pluralistic objection is to show that the non-Catholic view is as value-laden as any other.

Educating Health Care Providers about the *Directives*

The primary goal of health care ethics committees should be education—committee education and education of the institutional community. In the current climate of health care reform, the push for partnerships, and the promulgation of the *Directives* themselves, there exists a new and important opportunity for education in ethics. The *Directives* mandate the provision of "appropriate instruction regarding the directives for administration, medical and nursing staff and other personnel" (no. 5). The Pope John Center and the New England Chapter of the Catholic Health Association are currently engaged in a joint educational effort to explain the *Directives* to Catholic health care providers in New England with plans for other regions. The Catholic Health Association of the United States is giving its own presentations on the *Directives* as well. A concerted national effort to teach the new *Directives* might well be in order. Administrators and ethics committee chairmen would be aided in their efforts to educate their own institutions and committees by participating in workshops held across the country. On the committee level, planning could take place to reserve committee meeting time to learn about the *Directives* over the course of six months to a year. Institutionally, once the ethics committee members and other appropriate individuals are familiar with the *Directives*, they can present workshops, seminars, and orientation sessions on the *Directives* to the physician and nursing staffs. A similar sort of educational process might be advisable for Diocesan ethics committees. One timely tool for educating people about the *Directives* will be a manual for Catholic health care ethics committees currently being written by a Pope John Center task force which will include references to the *Directives*.

My final observation is that a most important element in any educational effort should be emphasis on the text of the *Directives*. As the Preamble notes, the *Ethical and Religious Directives for Catholic Health Care Services* is a document resulting from an extensive drafting process through which most of its words were carefully weighed, measured, and refined. The text should be the standard by which explanations of principles and cases are measured in educational programs about the *Directives*. The document will "mean what the words say" to quote Robert Bolt's Thomas More.[24] In a world where ethical issues are often decided according to a tyranny of words, the words of the *Ethical and Religious Directives for Catholic Health Care Services* will hopefully provide the anchor of meaning for caring with Christ's healing compassion.

Notes

1. Robert Bolt, *A Man for All Seasons* (New York: Vintage Books edition, 1990), 125.

2. *Ethical and Religious Directives for Catholic Health Care Services* (Washington, D.C.: United States Catholic Conference, 1995), 5.

3. Translated in *Vatican Council II: The Conciliar and Post Conciliar Documents*, General Editor, Austin Flannery, O.P. (Boston: St. Paul Editions, 1987).

4. National Conference of Catholic Bishops, "Resolution on Health Care Reform," *Origins*, vol. 23, no.7 (July 1, 1993): 101.

5. Jacques Maritain, *The Person and the Common Good*, translated by John J. Fitzgerald (Notre Dame: University of Notre Dame Press, 1966), 51-52.

6. *Directives*, p. 13.

7. Ibid., 13-14.

8. "Conscience and Truth" in *Catholic Conscience: Foundation and Formation*, ed. Russell E. Smith (Braintree, MA: The Pope John Center, 1991).

9. Ibid., 20.

10. Ibid.

11. Translation taken from Janet E. Smith, *Humanae Vitae: A Generation Later* (Washington: The Catholic University of America Press, 1991), 281.

12. The use of the terms "direct purpose" rather than "sole immediate effect" might prove to be too vague for a proper application of this Directive. "Direct purpose" is more susceptible to a subjective interpretation referring only to the subjective intentions of the agents.

13. See Peter J. Cataldo, "Anencephaly and Survivability," *Ethics & Medics*, vol. 18, no. 11 (November, 1993): 3-4.

14. The phrase, "to induce expectant mothers" appears in the cited section of *Donum Vitae*, but it is used strictly in the sense of condemning civil and health authorities or scientific organizations for *coercing* expectant mothers into having prenatal diagnosis for the purpose of elective abortion.

15. *Summa Theologica*, II-II, q. 65, a. 1, c. translated by the Fathers of the English Dominican Province (1911; rpt. Westminster, MD: Christian Classics, 1981).

16. *The Human Body*, selected and arranged by the Monks of Solesmes (Boston: St. Paul Editions, 1979), 198-199.

17. *Directives*, p. 21.

18. The correlativity of the obligations never to take innocent human life and to preserve life is evident in the exegesis of the commandment, "Thou shall not kill," by Pope John Paul II, in his encyclical, *Evangelium Vitae*: see nos. 40-41; 48; 54; and 75-76. The Pope shows the inextricable link between the two obligations and their

resulting equal moral status from the perspectives of their scriptural basis and from their internal logic. Throughout his analysis the Pope shows how the negative requirements of the commandment contain the positive requirements of respect for life. For example, from the scriptural perspective he writes: "By his words and actions Jesus further unveils the positive requirements of the commandment regarding the inviolability of life. These requirements were already present in the Old Testament..." (no. 41). The Pope shows how the commandment can actually become self-defeating if the inclusion of its positive requirement toward life is not recognized: "Detached from this wider framework, the commandment is destined to become nothing more than an obligation imposed from without, and very soon we begin to look for its limits and try to find mitigating factors and exceptions" (no. 48). The very nature of the absolute negative commandment entails a corresponding absolute positive requirement: "As explicitly formulated, the precept 'You shall not kill' is strongly negative: it indicated the extreme limit which can never be exceeded. Implicitly, however, it encourages a positive attitude of absolute respect for life" (54). What the commandment positively points and leads to is an absolute obligation: "For the Christian it [the commandment] involves an absolute imperative to respect, love and promote the life of every brother and sister..." (no. 77).

19. This concrete fulfillment of the obligation is reaffirmed in *Evangelium Vitae*, no. 65.

20. See *Summa Theologica*, I-II, q. 94, a. 2, c.

21. See *Evangelium Vitae*: "The commandment 'You shall not kill' thus establishes the point of departure for the start of true freedom. It leads us to promote life actively, and to develop particular ways of thinking and acting which serve life.... The commandment 'You shall not kill', even in its more positive aspects of respecting, loving and promoting human life, is binding on every individual human being" (nos. 76-77).

22. See *Directives*, p. 29.

23. *Ibid.*, 7.

24. Bolt, 125.

180

Chapter 12

RELIGIOUS LIBERTY
AND HEALTH CARE

Gerard V. Bradley, J. D.

My questions are two. First, to what extent will constitutional protections of religious liberty secure the autonomy that Catholic health care needs to remain faithful to the moral truth? Second, how does the answer to the first question affect the health—moral and physical—of our nation?

The matter is urgent. The need for autonomy is great; its prospects are doubtful. What might be called *de jure* heteronomy—state interference with the exercise of the Catholic health care apostolate—

is threatened by legal rights to immoral treatments, by public funding conditions which pressure providers to comply with patients' demands for them, and by potential malpractice liability for providers who do not cave in to the pressure.

A 1990 Fordham survey on Catholic institutional ministries tracked a steep decline in *de facto* autonomy.[1] The respondents included many Bishops. They noted that workers in Catholic health care are increasingly non-Catholic, and that these persons will need "special formation" for that Catholic ministry. The respondents thought that these ministries could serve non-Catholic clients and still be Catholic. But they anticipated that "empowerment" of the consumer would raise more of a "challenge" to Catholic identity in health care. It seems to me that the market presents the greatest threat to autonomy. Catholic health care faces the same pressures to enter mega-networks that secular hospitals do. But finding networks which permit Catholics to avoid all formal and unfair material cooperation in immoral acts is going to be very difficult.

That, all too briefly, is a sketch of the problem. Is the constitutional law of "religious liberty" the solution? I fear it is not. The constitutional law of religious liberty will undoubtedly secure autonomy in some instances, but not very many, and I am much inclined to think not enough to forestall the question of institutional martyrdom. That is basically because the constitutional law of religious liberty is more part of the threat to Catholic health care than it is part of a defense. The health of our society requires that we work to change our constitutional law of religious liberty.

Let me explain.

"Religious liberty," precisely so stated, does not appear anywhere in the Constitution. The relevant "constitutional protections" are the Religion Clauses of the First Amendment to the federal Constitution: the state shall pass no law "respecting an establishment of religion, or prohibiting the free exercise thereof." Authoritative judicial interpretation, the witness of history, and common sense hold that "religious liberty" is the aim of these clauses.

A preliminary clarification. For practical purposes the "Free Exercise" portion of "religious liberty" is supplied *not* by judicial construction of that constitutional provision. It is supplied by a statute. In a 1990 case[2] involving use of peyote in a native American religious ceremony, the Supreme Court gave what many said was a too-narrow reading of Free Exercise. In late 1993, President Clinton signed into law the Religious Freedom Restoration Act (RFRA).[3] It aimed to restore the assertedly broader understanding of Free Exercise which prevailed in the courts for a generation before the 1990 holding. This statute (RFRA) and the Establishment Clause are, for practical purposes, the relevant constitutional protections for religious liberty.

Let us start with RFRA. RFRA says that no "person"–defined elsewhere in the laws to include artificial persons like corporations as well as human individuals–may be "substantially burdened" in the exercise of religion, *unless* the law which imposes the substantial burden is "the least restrictive means" to furthering some "compelling governmental interest." This is basically a conscientious objection law and, seemingly, a strong one. The paradigm case might be the Jehovah's Witness who refuses to permit his child to receive a blood transfusion, when laws against child neglect would require it as a matter of parental duty. A parent who through simple neglect failed to order the transfusion would be arrested. A Jehovah's Witness likely would not be arrested, because his omission was no neglect of duty, but a response to a higher duty. Note that the practical effect of a successful invocation of RFRA is *not* to render a law unconstitutional. RFRA offers a special exemption for some specified persons from enforcement of what is assumed to be a valid and just law. So, relief sought by Catholic health care under RFRA would often not be sought under its proper description. The conscientious Catholic is often asserting a right not to be complicit in injustice, not a right of conscientious objection; the laws in question are themselves unjust, not just application to particular persons with odd views about morality. Abortion, suicide and the new reproductive technologies are examples.

RFRA's promise is to conscientious objectors only, and it is a shallow one. Consider RFRA's *indeterminacy*. Like the church-state corpus of which it is part, this is the jurisprudence of the adjective and the adverb: "substantially," "compelling," and "least restrictive" take their place alongside other critical terms of degree in church-state law: "primary" or "principal" effect, "excessive entanglement," and the like. The problem with these legal doctrines is like the problem with proportionalist moral absolutes. The so-called absolute *includes* an evaluative term. Do not "needlessly" kill the innocent, or "unjustifiably" commit adultery. The key moves remain hidden from view.

Which is to say that RFRA is transparent for judges with preanalytical convictions. These convictions are, by and large, much more like those of Jocelyn Elders and the dominant crew at the Cairo Conference than they are like those in this room. The elite culture's attitudes towards the morality of particular actions, and the elite culture's opinions of the Catholic Church, will very often have more to do with how cases come out than will legal doctrine.

A more straightforward problem with the "religious liberty" promised by RFRA is that it does not even address itself to *de facto* autonomy. RFRA considers exemption *only* from *government-imposed* "substantial burdens." Even then, courts have been unsympathetic to burdened plaintiffs. There have been just a handful of published opinions under RFRA (it has been law for just fifteen months), and no clear pattern of results has emerged, save that some prisoners denied regular opportunity to worship in unusual modes are faring well in court. But, prior to the 1990 case, the RFRA doctrine was applied many times, then as a construal of Free Exercise itself. I looked at, with a student's help, 100 random examples. In each, the plaintiff was a believer seeking relief from some burdensome law. In 94 out of 100, the courts *affirmed* government's right to burden the religious practice! This record, along with other evidence I have not the time to share, gives reason to wonder whether this doctrine of "religious liberty" is more a rhetorical campaign to justify coercion, than it is a genuine attempt to liberate religious conscience from legal burdens.[4]

Most important, the promise of RFRA is subordinate to the Establishment Clause. RFRA can only protect the free exercise of religion against "substantial" government burdens up to the point that such special consideration for religious believers runs into an Establishment Clause barrier. The Establishment Clause, in our law, trumps Free Exercise.

Where is *that* barrier? Let us consider first the history of it. The central command of the Establishment Clause was for a very long time rooted in the insight of the Founders that the common good of civil society did not depend upon the truth of the matters that distinguished the Protestant sects—finer points of doctrine, church discipline and polity, forms of worship. What distinguished Methodists from Presbyterians, the Founders concluded, could be safely declared beyond the competence of public authority. The law knew no heresy, no dogma, and established no sect.[5]

Now, this settlement *may* be inconsistent with *Dignitatus Humanae*. Whether it is inconsistent depends upon whether the obligation to recognize the true religion can be fulfilled by civil society, or whether it must include recognition of the true religion by the state. The latter prospect *is* definitely inconsistent with the fundamental positive law of *this* civil society, the Constitution.

But the Constitution was long understood in a way harmonious with *Dignitatus Humanae*: promoting the religious life of the people *was* permitted. It was commonplace. That all religions be treated equally—the doctrinal command that issued from the early insight—does not imply or provide an important premise for inferring that religion is something that is bad for persons or that it is something to be kept out of public life because dangerous to politics. "Religion" was not, by the way, Paul Tillich's "ultimate concern," but rather a community ordered around a particular way of being in communion with a greater than human source of meaning and value, which courts unashamedly called God. In this world, the rationale for promoting religious liberty was simple: religion was good. The state helped people to be good by helping them to be religious.

The central command of the Establishment Clause as interpreted by the Supreme Court since 1947 is this: public authority must not promote, encourage, foster, aid, or endorse religion, even if it would do so with a trace of partiality for one religion or another.[6] Why not? Because promoting or encouraging religion would violate the Supreme Court's command of neutrality. *This* neutrality is not between or among different faiths, but between religion and what the Court calls (but never defines as) "irreligion" or "nonreligion." A canonical expression: public authority may not favor "one religion over others nor religious adherents collectively over nonadherents."[7]

The Court's most recent (1994) case[8] presented a classic example of special care to assist believers to live out their commitments. The New York legislature carved out a village-sized school district to accommodate handicapped Hasidic Jewish children, who could not conscientiously go to public schools for the special education which federal statutes guaranteed them. (An aside: these children might otherwise have gone to private Jewish schools, and received their special ed services there. But this sensible solution was declared an unconstitutional establishment by the Supreme Court in 1985.[9])

The new accommodation was declared an unconstitutional establishment, too. Why? Because the Justices were not sure that the legislature would be "equally" solicitous of other "religious (and nonreligious) groups."[10] This same principle was expressed by Justice O'Connor in a concurring opinion: "Religious needs can [only!] be accommodated through laws that are neutral with regard to religion."[11] Otherwise, there would be prohibited "endorsement" of religion.

Make no mistake about it. This "superneutrality" controls the constitutional law of religious liberty. But here's the puzzle. Public authority *must*, according to RFRA, protect religious liberty. According to the Establishment Clause, however, public authority *may never* promote religion or take the view that religion is good. What coherent rationale then is there for "religious liberty"?

"Superneutrality" between belief and unbelief is, the Courts say, the mainstay, the stuff, of religious liberty. RFRA is about religious liberty. The question is: how can RFRA relieve burdens on "religion," in a way that does not discriminate in favor of religion over "nonreligion."

That Congress was puzzled about this may be evidenced from RFRA's nondefinition of religion: "exercise of religion," RFRA says, "means exercise of religion under the First Amendment to the Constitution."[12] That is, let the Courts solve the riddle they proposed back in 1947. One recent, self-conscious attempt to solve the riddle was Justice Souter's opinion (for O'Connor and Stevens) in a 1992 public school graduation prayer case, *Lee v. Wiseman.*[13] Souter wondered how state "accommodation" of burdens upon *just* the religious—basically, RFRA—*could be* consistent with the Establishment Clause. He opined that accommodation was all right because it showed only "respect" for *religion.* Souter said "respect" allows us to act "without expressing a position on the theological merit of those values."[14] Fair enough: we don't affirm the truth of some Islamic tenet when we say that Muslims have a right to "religious worship." Theirs is an exercise of religion, however theologically faulty it might be, and as an exercise of religion, has value. But Souter *then* claimed we "must respect" an exercise of religion without expressing a favorable view of "religious belief in general."[15] Souter is back where we began: on what basis do we act in some special way to "respect" *or* "accommodate" the "religious" practices of persons—what we seem to do --without "endorsing" religion, i.e., reject religion but *not* on the basis of *some* judgment about the value of religion?

"What makes accommodation permissible, even praiseworthy," Justice O'Connor said in the more recent Hasidim case, "is not that government is making life easier for some religious group as such. Rather, it is that government is accommodating a *deeply held belief.*"[16] Souter says, more revealingly: "in freeing the Native American Church from federal laws forbidding peyote use...the government conveys no endorsement of peyote rituals, the church, or *religion as such.* It simply respects the centrality of peyote to the lives of certain Americans."[17]

But *why* "certain" Americans, if *not* because Native American sacramental use has a value or is good in a way not present in non-sacramental uses? Clearly, the Justices are just *not* going to use the "R" word—religion—where the most obvious explanation for religious liberty would place it. This refusal to affirm religious goods as good has gotten hold of our law of religious liberty, and it won't let go.

What's happened is basically this. The law of religious liberty has been gobbled up by a wider civil liberty, the entirety of which is determined the moral subjectivism so powerfully criticized by the Pope in *Veritatis Splendor.* The Court began about three decades ago surrounding the subjectivist, sovereign self with impregnable constitutional defenses. On one flank the Justices upgraded moral decisions (like contraception, abortion) to the status of (without actually calling it) religion. In other words, they grounded pro-choice decisions in the "autonomy" of persons, glossed by a dreamy rhetoric of spiritual imperatives.

On the other flank, religion was downgraded from monotheism, in the 1950's, to any belief in God[s], to "ultimate concern," all the way to where belief and disbelief are now equally protected, self-defining choices. So the coherent rationale behind a "superneutrality" controlled religious liberty is that it's about liberty, *not* religion.

"Religious liberty" is, more exactly, about autonomy broadly understood as a private sphere in which everyone gets to do as they please so long as they visit no tangible harm upon nonconsenting third parties. In the eyes of the law, then, Billy Graham, Cardinal O'Connor, Shirley Maclaine, the village atheist, and people who express themselves by jitterbugging or listening to the Rolling Stones are all doing the same thing. They are doing *their* thing.

These developments were consummated in June 1992, in the Supreme Court decision which bears the name of the most courageous political figure in America. In what I call the "mystery passage" of *Planned Parenthood v. Casey*,[18] a plurality of Justices—Kennedy, O'Connor, Souter—spoke effectively for a majority. "At the heart of liberty is the right to define one's own concept of existence, of meaning, of the universe, and of the mystery of human life. Beliefs about these matters could not define the attributes of personhood were they formed under the compulsion of the state." [19] Thus, the State may not direct persons toward the good. The State must remain neutral about what constitutes genuine human flourishing.

Why is the "mystery" passage so important? Was it not, perhaps, an atypical statement, concocted as a way out of the abortion mess for some Justices with misgivings about *Roe*, but who were not prepared to reverse that infamous decision? Well, it *may* be that, but it is certainly a lot more. As the *Casey* joint opinion said, the "mystery passage" was the elusive (until then) rationale for a generation of important rulings in the areas of sexual morality, family life, education, and of course abortion.[20] The mystery passage, the Court meant, was the principle of *all* those decisions.

The mystery passage entailed, was a solution to the religious liberty dilemma. The dilemma, you recall, is how to make religious liberty equally available to the irreligious. *Casey* has the solution. Define religion in a way that includes everyone. Make "religion" out of existentially inevitable questions. Then everyone is religious, even atheists and agnostics.

Here's what *that* entails: not only are the woman giving birth and the woman down the hall aborting exercising the *same* constitutional right. According to *Casey* they most certainly are. The plurality dialectically defended the right to abort by saying that denying *it* would undermine the right to give birth.[21] It's worse than that: in light of *Lee v. Wiseman*, where Souter wondered about accommodated burdens, decided just five days before *Casey*, the priest baptizing the infant born, and the woman aborting, are exercising the exact same right—the right to "religious liberty," individual sovereignty over meaning, including the meaning of "good" and "evil."

I trust that few here will disagree that the sense has been entirely knocked out of the central presuppositions of our constitutional law. Religious liberty is smack in the middle of the contemporary autonomy project. That is what I meant when I said that it is part of the problem and not part of the solution: the *same* moral subjectivism that drives legal recognition (and funding) of objectively immoral treatments drives the law of religious liberty. In the new world of the autonomous self, Catholic doctors seeking the protective mantle of religious liberty will be seeking exemption *not* so much from laws serving "government interests" but from conflicting claims of patients to religious liberty—as defined by *Casey*. That is, once the courts have fully digested the *Casey* "mystery passage" and the moral subjectivism it harbors, the distinction between a "right" to religious liberty which trumps all but the most important government "interests" will fade. The suicide, and the Catholic physician trying to avoid assisting him, will be exercising precisely the same right to fathom the mysteries of the universe. They will both be exercising autonomy, in the so-called private sphere, trying not to visit harm upon each other.

What then is to be done?

I do not counsel shunning the courts. I do not think it immoral in itself, or otherwise imprudent, for Catholic hospitals to sue under RFRA to gain some measure of autonomy. They might win, and asserting one's legal rights, where the sense of the law—but not the specific legal doctrine being relied upon—is twisted, is neither immoral in itself nor scandalous.

But Catholic health care will more often lose in court. Besides the limitations of RFRA I have mentioned, is this new megaright of persons to be let alone, to let everyone do his thing, short of tangible harm to others? This aspiration is not commodious enough to provide all the room that the norms require against culpable cooperation and giving scandal, as well as the affirmative duty of any Catholic apostolate to give clear and consistent witness. More exactly: Catholics don't want to be left alone; they are committed to moral truth, and to serving the common good. Besides, due to simple muddleheadedness, and to judicial efforts to pour the new wine of autonomy into the old wineskins of traditional morality, courts are ill prepared to really understand what it would mean for Catholics to really enjoy autonomy. Two examples: in *law*, the pill and the IUD, which work in truth sometimes as abortifacients, are deemed "contraceptives." Autonomy granted on abortion—a plausible scenario—therefore will *not* extend to the IUD. Also, judges hostile to a right to assisted suicide have this in common with judges who think persons have a right to kill themselves: they brand as "letting die" or "nature taking its course" many acts which are choices to kill oneself, reflective of judgments that life is sometimes an evil, that death is sometimes a good which may, *as such*, be chosen. Suicide, by any other name, is still suicide. In some of these cases the grasp of what distinguishes an act for moral evaluative purposes—what the Holy Father so lucidly discusses in *Veritatis Splendor* (no. 78)—is so loose that the judge would be unable to distinguish the martyr's death, or Jesus' crucifixion, from a suicide. Thus, courts inclined to exempt Catholic doctors from complicity in killing—at each end of life—will be erratic allies. They simply do not know what killing *is*.

It seems to me that so long as the prevailing approach to "religious liberty" obtains, there is virtually no chance of survival for Catholic health care. The subjectivism which has taken over the law will generate new demands for objectively immoral treatments very rapidly. Even if the legal system, including "religious liberty" guarantees, shelters us on, say, abortion, it is unlikely to allow clearheaded and conscientious Catholics the room they need to avoid all formal and unfair material cooperation in contraception, including so-called contraceptives like IUD. If I am wrong about *that*, within a very short time Catholics will very likely be faced with challenges to conscience by assisted suicide (called by the law "letting die"). Shortly after that, "genetic counseling" and "genetic engineering" are liable to be standard practice in medicine. The prospect in a decade or two of "designer babies" may well be too much for most people to resist. You get the idea. My point: *success on each and every one of these fronts is necessary to avoid institutional martyrdom*. It is not enough to preserve "Catholic identity," to have clean hands on say sterilizations and abortions, but to be complicit in suicide. We need to bat one thousand percent in this league.

There seems to be no alternative to institutional martyrdom, other than taking on the prevailing view itself. The moral health of our nation requires no less. (An aside: I suppose that martyred Catholic hospitals will be taken over by secular managers. In a certain way, then, the physical health of the nation is not at stake.)

Where do we start taking on the prevailing view? There are two pressure points you might attend, one specifically constitutional, the other a more general piece of advice for a political strategy. Litigation should focus on reversing the determining feature of all our Church-State doctrine: the "no-aid" principle and its resulting "neutrality" between religion and irreligion. There are now *three* votes on the Supreme Court—Thomas, Scalia, Rehnquist—for this reversal. Justice Kennedy is perplexed, and might still go with Scalia, et al. Depending on the outcome of the next Presidential election, it may not be at all naive to think that the necessary vote (or two) could be added. This part of church-state doctrine is the linchpin, so to speak, of the entire autonomy project of the last thirty years or so. Make *it* a "litmus test," if you will, of any nominee to the Supreme Court.

The broader point has to do with the central aspiration of the autonomy project, especially as instantiated in the Church-State corpus: public authority must do nothing that "alienates" someone and thereby puts him or her into an "outsider" group of "second class" citizens. I submit that it is impossible to overstate the importance of this aspect, captured by so many sound bites in our political culture: "neutrality," "inclusiveness," "divisiveness," and a potpourri of egalitarian themes. The contemporary state is very worried about religious believers who might wonder about whether the common good is really the principle of their government actions, after all.

I propose that the American Catholic community register, in the most profound way, its doubts about whether we can be "insiders." John Courtney Murray set the precedent here, in his famous essay on civil unity.[22] Murray reviewed the history and jurisprudence of the Religion Clauses, and noted several interpretations then in the air which were flatly incompatible with Catholics' commitment to the regime. Look it up. Murray laid down the challenge in stark terms: there will be, he said, immediately some 35 million dissenters—the Roman Catholic community—in this country if certain interpretations of the First Amendment are adopted. One of them has in effect been adopted. Now, there are 60 million Roman Catholics in America. If they—or even very many of them—speak out against the new subjectivism, they can probably change the culture. I fear that they will have to speak out, *if* Catholic health care is to survive.

Notes

1. C. Fahey, et al., editors, *The Future of Catholic Institutional Ministries* (Bronx, N.Y.: Third Age Center, Fordham University, 1992).

2. Oregon v. Smith, 494 U.S. 8782 (1990).

3. 42 U.S.C. 2000 bb (1993).

4. See G. Bradley, "Beguiled: Free Exercise Exemptions and the Siren Song of Liberalism," *Hofstra Law Review* 20 (1991): 245, 307-19.

5. See generally "Beguiled," *supra* note 4, and G. Bradley, *Church-State Relationships in America* (New York: Greenwood Press, 1987).

6. See Everson v. Board of Education, 330 U.S. 1 (1947).

7. Kiryas Joel v. Grumet, 114 S.Ct. 2481, 2487 (1994).

8. Kiryas Joel, supra note 7.

9. Aguilar v. Felton, 473 U.S. 402 (1985).

10. 114 *S.Ct.* at 2491.

11. 114 *S.Ct.* at 2496.

12. RFRA, § 5(4).

13. 112 S.Ct. 2649 (1992).

14. 112 S. Ct. at 2677.

15. Id.

16. 114 S. Ct. at 2497 (my emphasis).

17. 112 S. Ct. at 2649.

18. 112 S. Ct. 2791 (1992).

19. 112 S. Ct. at 2807.

20. Id.

21. "If indeed the woman's interest in deciding whether to bear and beget a child had not been recognized as in *Roe*, the State might as readily restrict a woman's right to choose to carry a pregnancy to term as to terminate it, to further asserted state interests in population control, or eugenics, for example." 112 S. Ct. at 2811.

22. J. Murray, *We Hold These Truths* (New York: Sheed and Ward, 1960), 45-78.

Chapter 13

PUBLIC POLICY AND MORAL TRUTH

The Honorable Robert P. Casey

Today's topic, "Public Policy and Moral Truth," sounds very abstract and philosophical. But I want to begin with something very immediate and tangible, some images from the news that I've been turning over in my mind lately. Ethical questions do not, after all, arise in a void. So before discussing the obligations of public persons from my personal perspective, I will offer some observations about world opinion and what I see as its significance today.

One image comes to us from the other side of the world. All of you, I'm sure, saw the same news accounts I did from Pope John Paul's recent trip to the Philippines. You saw the same pictures–to my mind, amazing pictures. Here was the leader of our Church; a Church that, so many of these same newspapers remind us again and again on other occasions, has grown "narrow" in outlook, "estranged" from popular opinion.

But look at the audience: Somewhere from four to five million people came out one day to greet him. *Four to five million people.* That's an awful lot of people for a church that's getting more narrow in outlook.

Meanwhile, as all of us know, the Pope has published a book. Not an encyclical addressed only to Catholics, but a book for anyone who cares to read it, a book addressed to the world. And to judge by sales, it turns out the world is interested. At the same time, in the record stores no item is moving faster today than a recording of John Paul II praying the rosary—in Latin.

What marketing executive would have told you the Rosary could ever top the charts? But there it is—the most popular recording in the world today.

Who's buying the recording and reading the book? It would be easy to say that for the most part older Catholics account for this commercial smash. But there's a problem with that explanation: In Manila, the occasion was Youth Day. And closer to home, what about the 350,000 teenagers who turned out for Youth Day last year when the Pope came to Denver?

Again, news commentary strained to explain it all by the sheer celebrity of the Pope. He's famous, a "star," so that must explain the big turnout. Well, that's not the impression I had. Let's try another explanation. I remember in particular the quote of one 17-year-old young woman: "There aren't many leaders around today," she said. "But this man—he's a leader." And the young woman, according to the story, was not a Catholic. Another young woman said this to a reporter: "I don't react this way to rock groups. What is it that he has?"

To top it all off, you pick up *Time* magazine, and there he is again, the "Man of the Year"—Pope John Paul II. Only this past fall, we heard warnings that his firm pro-life stance at the Cairo conference on population threatened to render the Church irrelevant in world opinion. The train of history was pulling out of Cairo, and John Paul was about to miss it. The Catholic Church would defy Vice President Gore and the population control advocates at its peril.

But now, only four months later, it's pretty clear who had the wrong train schedule.

Apparently, John Paul knows more about world opinion than they gave him credit for. Listen to how *Time* put it: "It is…with increased urgency that John Paul has presented himself, the defender of Roman Catholic doctrine, as a moral compass for believers and nonbelievers alike. He spread through every means at his disposal a message not of expedience or compromise but of right and wrong; amid so much fear of the future, John Paul dared to speak of hope…."

His goals, said *Time*, are grand, "informed by a vision as vast as the human determination to bring them into being. After discovering the principle of the lever and the fulcrum in the Third Century B.C., Archimedes wrote, 'Give me a place to stand, and I will move the earth'. John Paul knows where he stands."

As Catholics in the year 1995, we are blessed to know where we stand. We are blessed to be under the guidance of a true leader of men; a man whose whole being points the way. So often over the past 16 years, he has been offered the world in exchange for one favor. I think of it as a modern reenactment of the temptation in the wilderness: If only you will do one thing for me, says the world, I will give you all this. Compromise just this once, qualify by just one shade this belief in the sanctity of life—and we'll praise your name. We'll accept you. But he never has, and look at the results. Show me a more revered figure today. Show me someone else who can draw five million people by his mere presence. Show me a person who commands more of the world's respect and attention.

Bearing these images in mind, the whole question of reconciling public duty with private conscience takes on real life. It is not a part of some dry academic debate; it is a matter of the most profound urgency. John Paul is a spiritual leader, but reflected in those crowds is, I believe, something of which every public official had better take note. This is the world in which a political leader today faces his responsibilities. And with those obligations, his opportunities. These are the people he or she would lead. It is a world distrustful of secular visions, a world deeply wary of moral compromise. They—we—are a people yearning for moral leadership.

I read something recently that speaks directly to this moral deficit and our role as Catholics in setting it right. It was an essay by a very distinguished person whom I have had the good fortune to meet, Father William Miscamble of Notre Dame. He issued a challenge, a call really, for political courage. "Those Catholics," he wrote, "who believe their church's teachings—on respect for human life, on concern for the common good, on responsibilities as well as individual rights...have something important to contribute to American political life."

That call, if anything, understates the case. We not only have something important to contribute. With other people of faith, we have something absolutely essential; something for which America is waiting; something without which it may not survive.

Are there limitations to what the man or woman of faith can accomplish in politics? Sure there are. Always have been. Whatever dilemmas there might be in political life, they are by no means new to our day. Any man who has ever tried to use political power for the common good has felt an awful sense of powerlessness. There are always limits to what we can do, always obstacles, always frustrations and bitter disappointments.

This was the drama a future president once studied in *Profiles in Courage*, a book that now seems quaint in its simple moral idealism. The founders of our country understood the limits of political power when they swore allegiance to something higher, their "sacred honor." Lincoln felt this tension when he sought to uphold the equality of men. Likewise, Thomas More expressed the dilemma when, faced with the raw power of the state, he declared: "I die the king's good servant but God's first." Far from being a new problem, this tension goes all the way back to the Pharisees and their challenge to declare for or against Caesar.

But, less profoundly, I would point out one thing about the tensions and dilemmas of political life. They are tensions merely between effort and expectation. The fact that we can never attain a perfect world does not relieve us of the duty to fight for a more just world. Otherwise, the fight would never have to be taken up in the first place; we could all in perfectly good conscience sit around and do nothing. All these well-known dilemmas are an argument for prudence, not for pragmatism; for determination, not despair. They are not an invitation to capitulation. They are not an excuse for the timid.

We have all heard fellow Catholics agonizing over the dilemmas of public life, as if private conscience and public conduct presented some inherent conflict, as if you have two consciences, one for work and one for home.

I will not disparage this view except to say that as governor of a highly diverse state, I was always struck by just the opposite: the remarkable convergence between the general principles of our faith and the ideas of justice that shaped this nation. Merely to recite the teachings Father Miscamble mentions calls to mind the whole experience of the American people.

We are, first and foremost, the country described in our birth certificate, the Declaration of Independence. We're a nation born of the conviction that all are created equal in rights and dignity. America began with that one brave assertion of truth, a truth for all people in all times. In that truth lies our national calling, our compact, our destiny.

Sure, at other times religious influence had been excessive, overbearing. Why has American history been different? Not, I believe, because religious and moral belief was banished from the public square—quite the contrary—but because conscience was welcomed. Call these religious convictions, call them moral values, call them points of natural law. But whatever we call them, they are not narrow, divisive ideas. They are the ideas that from the very start have kept us together as a people. Always we have been a people to whom religion and morality have been as vital, essential, and ever-present as the air we breathe. If there is any common thread to the American story, this is it: A diversity of beliefs, but a unity in moral purpose, a coming together in conscience.

If, for example, the question is, "Do we protect the most vulnerable in our society?" then let me just admit it outright—the dilemma eludes me. My faith, my conscience, my political philosophy, and my nation's credo all speak with one voice. The times may change; one party may fall and another prevail; the next election may be tomorrow or four years from now. But through it all my basic obligations remain the same. Conscience remains "the still point in the turning wheel."

Often in our political debates, I think of a line spoken by Thomas More in the play *A Man for All Seasons*. "I believe," he says, "when statesmen forsake their own private consciences for the sake of their public duties...they lead their country by a short route to chaos."

Perhaps never in history has the route been shorter than in the painful journey we began with *Roe v. Wade*. Here, more than anywhere, the voice of conscience comes to me resoundingly. When the question is, "Do we as a society have a compelling interest in the fate of the unborn? Do we love them or consent to their destruction?"—reason, natural law, our religious traditions and centuries of jurisprudence speak as one.

Today, we see in the national liberal and conservative policies of our country a temptation to ignore the serious demands of conscience: to abdicate responsibilities for others and acquiesce in a breakdown of our sense of community, the common good, and respect for human life.

Both ends of the philosophical spectrum tend to fall prey to a different set of temptations.

On the one hand, many conservatives seem to close their eyes to the common good and the societal obligation to the less fortunate, the sick, the poor, the unemployed, the homeless, to all of those who need a helping hand.

And yet for Catholics, this challenge of finding a true social responsibility still stands. The obligation is spelled out clearly, from *Rerum Novarum* of Leo XIII to *Solicitudo Rei Socialis* of John Paul II. The Church's teaching has consistently stressed the obligation to work for social justice and the common good, by fighting for life and balancing rights with responsibilities, working to strengthen family and community, and helping the poor. And I am clear that, as part of this societal response, government has a necessary role to play.

As Governor of Pennsylvania, I have tried to meet this challenge. Because adequate health care is a right, I have set up health care programs for women and children that have been called a model for the nation. Because our concern for the poor should increase rather than decrease when times are hard, I refused to cut welfare benefits for women, children, and families during the recent recession. And in the current national debate on welfare reform, we should oppose public policies like the so-called family cap, which denies benefits to women who have additional children, because they have the effect of taking food from the mouths of innocent children and providing incentives to increase the number of abortions in this country. In Pennsylvania, I started a health insurance program for poor children, and have made adoption a statewide priority, and most important, we have passed the nation's strongest laws protecting unborn children.

So much for the conservative side of the spectrum. When you look at the liberal side, there are deficiencies just as serious. There we see a breakdown in responsibility and community and an excessive emphasis on rights to the exclusion of corresponding responsibilities.

License is favored over true liberty, which is the freedom to do what we ought to do. Relativism is rampant, ignoring the fundamental and changeless absolute that there always have been, there are now, and there always will be, things that are right, and things that are wrong. Support for the liberal social justice agenda should not carry with it an open-ended endorsement of the liberal cultural agenda which runs contrary to our most basic values.

Liberals speak of the "quality of life" ethic to justify abortion. A child, if born, will face hardship; therefore, destroy it. A baby will only burden one's personal economic situation, or require public assistance, or cause inconvenience all around; therefore, do everyone the favor of aborting it. Get rid of it and all will be well. This may be putting it harshly, but that in the end is how this reasoning operates.

As a Democrat of long standing, when people start using phrases like "quality of life," I hear echoes of the "rugged individualism" of another era. At the heart of both, it seems to me, is a worship of the self; self-love instead of love for others. In both we hear the same knack for casting raw self-interest in the language of altruism. Both are visions of power, not love, as the highest human achievement.

As a nation, we are seeing the fruits of the false and empty promises of liberation held out by abortion on demand and no-fault divorce. These include the increasing feminization of poverty and family disintegration.

And so, we see these twin tendencies at work: an indifference to private responsibility on the one hand, and an indifference to social responsibility on the other. Their advocates seem to be saying that as a society we cannot do any better than just simply leaving each other alone. But that is not the American experience. I believe America is better than that. I know America is better than that. And our history confirms it.

In concluding, let me go back to the image of Pope John Paul II and the hope he represents. Sometimes Christians are tempted to take a discouraged, downcast view of the modern world. Sometimes these views have bordered on a despair for America that I myself do not share. Maybe the best description was offered 50 years ago by the Scottish author John Buchan. Even then, he could see "the coming of a too garish age, when life would be lived under the glare of neon lamps and the spirit would have no place for solitude." In such a world, he said:

> ...everyone would have leisure. But everyone would be restless for there would be no spiritual discipline in life.... It would be a feverish, bustling world, self-satisfied and yet malcontent, and under the mask of a righteous life there would be death at the heart. In the perpetual hurry of life there would be no quiet for the soul. [In such a world] life would be rationalized and padded with every material comfort, [but] there would be little satisfaction for the immortal part of man.

But here, I believe, is what we have to understand: As true a picture as this may be, it is an incomplete picture of modern society in 1995. It is a still shot, one frame in a social and spiritual drama that is moving quickly. You'd have to be sleepwalking through the world to miss what's happening: We have put our faith in things that failed us, and the disappointment is deep and bitter.

Something big—almost too big to comprehend—is underway, not only in America, but the world over. In developed nations, the people have filled themselves with all that modern life can provide. And they've been left empty. Most of them for half a century have enjoyed greater personal freedom. But even that has left them unfulfilled, and in some ways less free. In the abortion culture, we walked away from an entire class of humanity. But still we look back. And now, I believe, we are turning back, and turning back we see what else we left behind: our national soul, our common mission, our vision of who we are.

I have heard even his admirers say of John Paul: He stands out only because "the light shines brighter in the darkness"; because he is the last of his kind, the last gasp of a passing moral order. And I don't, for one moment, believe it. On the contrary, just the opposite is true. I believe he stands for a new beginning and not an end—the future, not the past. He shines only because people are ready to catch his reflection. His voice resonates because he offers something better. Wherever his message goes, millions come in hope of receiving it.

In our politics, something similar is unfolding. Those who offer only material cures to our troubles seem almost pathetically irrelevant. They are destined to be swept away. Those cures have been tried. Sometimes they have been successful, sometimes not. Legitimate debates are now under way as to what material aid government should provide. I know where I come down on the question: Through government, we must always care for the weak and vulnerable.

But on one point there is an emerging consensus: no purely material or financial vision of public leadership can ever answer our deepest need. We are not just ciphers of the state awaiting government direction; and neither are we just consumers, each making a little contribution to private profits and the GNP. We are people of greater vision than that. Each one of us has a spiritual calling that reaches into our common life together. We have passed through that age of garish things and feverish pursuits and hollow satisfactions. Certain features of it remain and probably will remain for some time to come. But if we look around, the signs are everywhere that as a people, we hear our true calling. We search for something better. The only question is how clearly our leaders hear that same call, and whether they have the courage to rise to it.

In the context of abortion, the truth about human dignity, justice, and social responsibility clearly represents a grave, historic challenge for us and for the entire nation. It is telling that the new *Catechism* speaks about abortion not in terms of the moral demands on individuals, but entirely in terms of the responsibility of society to protect unborn human life. Speaking of abortion, Pope John Paul II's new book calls for "radical solidarity with the woman."

We must make our voices heard, speak the truth fearlessly, and act decisively in both the personal and the political spheres on behalf of both mother and child, before and after birth. If we are not to present a distorted version of our message, we must refuse to compromise either our active compassion or our steadfast principles.

In responding to the challenge, we must follow the example of John Paul. We must dare to speak of hope. We must dare to believe in ourselves—in the common sense and basic goodness of the American people.

There is no need to wait for a "consensus." Leaders do not wait for a consensus; they inspire one. And, my friends, that consensus is here. It was formed when as a nation we looked at the alternative to faith and saw a terrifying void, a short road to chaos, a vision of power alone untempered by love. In the cause of life, the consensus is profound; it grows every time someone looks at a sonogram. Joining it by the day are people unafraid of criticism and derision; people with eyes to see, a mind to reason, and a heart to feel.

All we need are leaders. Not apologists to soothe us into inaction. We don't need more people to diagnose the problem, to agonize over the problem, to ponder the odds of overcoming the problem. We need leaders, moral leaders, to work for change.

I know we can count on the spiritual leadership of the Pope and the Bishops—all of those gathered here today and those who could not be here. In the face of tremendous hostility and adversity, you have been stalwart witnesses, courageous champions of the truth.

But what we need above all today are leaders in medicine, journalism, law, and government. Leaders who will take seriously the compelling challenge to offer their witness in the public square. Leaders with a strong dimension of generosity and understanding, sending a message of civility and respect for opposing views, a message that bespeaks a true sense of community. Leaders who condemn violence whenever and wherever it appears. Leaders who present the protection of the unborn child from what it truly is—an imperative that flows naturally from the historic social justice mission of America.

Leaders who will stand firmly on the ground of hope, and, with the lever of truth, move the world.

Chapter 14

A CATHOLIC PERSPECTIVE ON HEALTH CARE POLICY

The Most Reverend John H. Ricard, S.S.J.

I am honored by the invitation to address this important topic at this distinguished gathering. When this invitation was first issued, health care reform was the dominant political issue before the nation. I'm tempted to address the moral dimensions of welfare reform (the issue of the moment), but I won't. Health care may have moved from the center of American politics and policy, but it remains a vital, if less visible, concern for our people. And it continues to be a major priority and commitment for our Catholic community of faith. Our

Church brings a long history of ethical reflection, day-to-day experience, and public advocacy to health care policy. These strengths remain valuable assets in the current health care environment.

As I begin, I feel the need to offer a few caveats regarding my assignment today. In light of the dramatically different political climate, I will focus less on the specifics of a possible benefit package and more on the broader ethical principles which should shape health policy. While I am honored to be a part of this gathering, I am, like you, a bishop. I am a pastor, not a public policy worker; a teacher, not a health technician. My reflections today are drawn primarily from my ministry as a pastor in poor parishes in both Baltimore and Washington and my past experience as a counselor and social worker in these communities. They also reflect my current responsibilities as Chairman of the Domestic Policy Committee of the U.S. Bishops' Conference, which has a lead responsibility in the area of health care reform. We closely coordinate our efforts with other committees who also have vital roles in this area (e.g., Pro-life, Doctrine, Migration, Hispanic and African American).

This is not a new concern for our Church. Seventy-five years ago, the American Catholic bishops declared, "The state should make comprehensive provision for insurance against illness..." Throughout this century, the bishops have urged health care reform. Eighteen months ago, we unanimously adopted a major resolution to guide our approach to health care reform. As you know all too well, a unanimous vote is an unusual achievement for our Conference. It reflects a broad consensus among the bishops. Today, I wish to revisit the basic principles of that resolution and offer some thoughts on three related areas:

—Lessons Learned from Last Year's Debate
—The Ongoing Problems in Health Care
—The Principles, Priorities and Potential of the Catholic Community in Health Care.

I
Lessons Learned

Let me begin with some of the lessons of last year's health care reform debate. As you all know, despite high expectations and considerable sound and fury, the Congress failed to seriously debate, much less enact, comprehensive health care reform legislation. This was the result of a combination of weak political leadership, partisan conflict, special interest pressures and substantial public doubts about government's capacity and competence in health care.

The debate was much more soundbites and attack ads than civil dialogue and the search for the common good. The Administration produced an extraordinarily complicated proposal without broad or bipartisan support, flawed in both process and product and burdened by particular special interest provisions (i.e., abortion mandates). Most Republican legislators in the end decided their political needs would best be served by determined opposition more than constructive compromise. Powerful interests mobilized their financial and political resources to block any reform that threatened their part of the status quo. And the public was left confused and divided, with deep conflicts over the role of government, employers, and individuals in health care and fearful that political leaders would do more harm than good.

Many people were looking for painless reform. They hope to pay less for more care. They hope to assure health care access and security for all without greater sacrifices, increased taxes, or diminished choices for anyone.

The illusions of painless reform will eventually have to yield to the hard choices of how to expand access, how to restrain costs, and who pays. Each of these choices has major ethical dimensions. They reflect values of human life and human dignity, questions of distributive justice and subsidiarity, and priorities in allocating benefits and burdens. They go to the heart of what kind of society we are and will be, the value we place on human life, and how we treat the weak and vulnerable, sick and suffering. We are still faced with this question: "Are we prepared to make the changes, address the neglect, accept the sacrifices, and practice the discipline that can lead to better health care for all Americans?"

I believe last year's debate did not do justice to the issue or serve the nation. Across the spectrum, politics prevailed over substance, narrow interests over the common good. The nation has yet to really face the challenge of health care reform.

The health care debate did not enrich the nation, but it brought major elements of our Church together. It seems to me the Catholic community did a better job on health care reform than the Congress. Our Bishops' Conference offered strong, united advocacy on behalf of both the unborn and the unserved. Our approach focused on advancing our principles and priorities, not on advocating specific proposals. Our message of no to abortion mandates and yes to universal coverage clearly reflected our tradition and teaching. We didn't choose between our priorities, but fought for both. A few in the Catholic community objected to one or the other of our priorities, but I believe they brought unity, credibility, and consistency to our efforts.

The intense collaboration in our Conference and in dioceses helped us carry this message forward. While I'm Chairman of the Domestic Committee, I seemed to spend most of my time making the case in the media and on Capitol Hill against abortion mandates. Cardinal Mahony is Chairman of the Pro-life Committee, but he is one of the strongest supporters of universal coverage. And the grass-roots advocacy was unprecedented—millions of post cards; countless letters, homilies and bulletin inserts; hundreds of columns and ads; and an impressive number of face to face and telephone visits with legislators. I want to thank the many bishops who responded to our appeals for help.

The Catholic community was seen as a serious, principled, and involved constituency on health care. But the combination of partisan conflict, special interest pressure, and lack of consensus on the basics ultimately led to political stalemate and a failure of Congress to act.

I believe we have laid the groundwork for *future* Catholic advocacy on health care which protects human life and advances human dignity. I believe consistent commitment to principle continues to offer the best path for the future. Just as we did not abandon the unborn when a new Administration came to power, we cannot abandon the uninsured and undocumented when a new majority takes control of Congress. We must find effective ways to advance old values in a new political climate, but we cannot walk away from our teaching or those who lack adequate health care.

II
The Continuing Problems

The last point is important because the problems are not going away. The nation's health care situation can still be summed up in one sentence—our health care system serves too few and costs too much. In many respects we have the best health care in the world, with remarkable medical technology, institutions, and professionals. But 37 million Americans lack effective access to our health care system, including 10 million children. It is estimated that 100,000 people lose their health care coverage each month.

This means one in six Americans does not have health care coverage. This figure has gone up six million over the last five years. Seventy-five percent of those without coverage are full time workers and their children—a surprising statistic since many Americans believe the uninsured are mostly poor and unemployed. The lack of coverage matters; babies born into families without insurance are 30% more likely to die or be seriously ill at birth.

In addition, the burdens of our system are not shared equally: one in five African Americans lacks insurance; one in three Hispanics; and one in ten white Americans. While infant mortality went down last year, we still rank behind most industrialized countries, and in our inner cities the infant mortality rates approach Third World levels. African American babies are twice as likely as white babies to die in their first year.

There also continues to be an erosion of employer sponsored health insurance. In 1988, 62% of Americans got their insurance through their employment. In 1993, that number had decreased to 57%.

So lack of access remains a central priority. No industrialized country has so many people without regular access to care. This fact has significant human consequences and ethical implications.

A second continuing problem is rapidly rising health care costs which are seriously impacting the nation's economy, family budgets, government deficits, business finances, and religious institutions. At current rates of inflation, it is estimated that health care costs are headed for two trillion dollars by the year 2000—more than triple what they were in 1990.

Although some have applauded the recent slowdown in health care inflation, health care prices are still rising twice as fast as the general price level. In the last two years, health prices have risen at about a 5% annual rate, while overall consumer prices have risen at a 2.6% rate.

We pay far more for health care than other industrial countries. Health care is now the most common cause of labor disputes and a factor in half of this nation's bankruptcies. The emphasis on high-tech medicine, the focus on acute care rather than prevention, waste and duplication, the aging of our population, and lack of fiscal accountability have produced surging health care inflation. This inflation not only makes health care unaffordable for many, but leaves fewer and fewer resources for education, job creation, housing, and other national needs.

Because of these two fundamental problems—lack of access and rising costs—and the continuing threat that even incremental reform may include a basic benefits package mandating abortion coverage, health care policy remains a continuing concern of our Bishops' Conference. Health care reform may not be a pressing political priority for the nation at this moment. It was not even mentioned in the Republican "Contract with America." But it will continue to be an important policy issue because the nation's health problems will not be addressed without real reform. That reform is likely to be incremental, rather than comprehensive; but the status quo is already giving way to a new health care environment, and reform will come.

The future debate and decisions will not be easy. They will touch every family and business, every community and parish; health care represents a seventh of our national economy. I believe this issue will continue to test our nation and challenge our Church.

III
The Principles, Priorities and Potential of the Catholic Community in Health Care

I believe no community has more at stake or more to contribute to this continuing process than the Catholic community. At the outset, it is important to remind ourselves we are a community of faith, not a political interest group. In Washington, the battle over health care reform was driven by political resources we don't possess. Campaign contributions, high priced lobbyists, attack commercials, and partisan gamesmanship, thankfully, are not a part of Catholic advocacy on health care. We bring a different set of assets which, I believe, over time can help make the case for necessary reform. Let me mention three particular resources we bring: strong convictions, broad experience, and a capacity for advocacy.

A. First, we bring to this debate a set of *fundamental values and principles*. We have in the scriptures and Catholic Social Teaching key values and principles to guide our health care advocacy. We don't redefine ourselves according to the opinion polls or latest election results. Let me cite four key principles:

1. The first value is a *consistent commitment to human life and human dignity*. In our tradition, the human person is central. We measure every policy or proposal by whether it protects or threatens human life, whether it enhances or undermines human dignity. Our Church teaches that every person has the right to life and those things which protect and sustain life, including and especially health care. In the words of *Pacem in Terris*:

   Every man has the right to life, to bodily integrity, and to the means which are suitable for the proper development of life; these are primarily food, clothing, shelter, rest, medical care, and finally the necessary social services. Therefore a human being also has the right to security in cases of sickness, inability to work, etc.[1]

In our tradition, health care is not a product or commodity—it is an essential safeguard of human life and dignity. We believe a person's health care should not depend on where they work, how much their parents earn, or where they live. When millions of Americans are without health coverage, when rising costs threaten the coverage of millions more, when infant mortality remains shockingly high, the right to health care is seriously undermined and our health care system is in need of fundamental reform.

2. A second value is our *option for the poor and vulnerable.* We are called to measure a society by how it treats the weak and powerless. We look at health care from the bottom up. For us, the key criteria for health care policy is not how it treats the doctors or insurance companies, the well-off and powerful, but how it serves the poor and the unserved, the unborn and the undocumented. As Pope John Paul II said in *Centesimus Annus*:

> When there is question of defending the rights of individuals, the defenseless and the poor have a claim to special consideration. The richer class has many ways of shielding itself, and stands less in need of help from the State; whereas the mass of the poor have no resources of their own to fall back on, and must chiefly depend on the assistance of the State.[2]...there are many human needs which find no place on the market. It is a strict duty of justice and truth not to allow fundamental human needs to remain unsatisfied, and not to allow those burdened by such needs to perish.[3]

3. A third value is the traditional principle of *stewardship.* We recognize there are limits on our national resources and we know the impact of rapidly rising costs of health care. Our nation is morally required to address the waste, duplication, and unrestrained costs of our system and its impact on individuals, families, institutions, and the entire society. Stewardship demands effective efforts to restrain rising costs.

4. A fourth value is the principle of the *common good.* In the midst of the partisan battles, and the inevitable clash of powerful economic interests, we believe the basic test will be how health care policy serves the good of the whole nation, not the narrow interests of the powerful or partisan needs of politicians.

There are other principles which could be cited (i.e., the responsibility and limitations of government, subsidiarity, and solidarity) and people of good faith and good will can disagree on how they are to be applied, but I believe these four are useful foundations for an ethical evaluation of health policy. They help the Catholic community bring a moral perspective in an intensely political debate, offer an ethical framework in an arena dominated by major institutional interests.

B. A second major asset we bring is *broad experience* in health care. We bring not only strong convictions, but also a long history and everyday experience in this area. Aside from government itself, no institution in American life is more involved in so many aspects of health care.

The Catholic Community is a *major provider* of health care. Religious communities and dioceses operate 600 hospitals, 300 long term facilities, and hundreds of clinics and other health ministries. We are the largest non-profit provider of health care, serving tens of millions of patients each year.

We are also a *major purchaser* of health care. Catholic institutions provide health care coverage for hundreds of thousands of employees and their families. Our ministry and programs are squeezed and our services reduced because of the rapidly rising costs of health care.

We are also a community that *picks up the pieces* of a failing health care system. The children without care, the families without insurance, the sick without options are in our emergency rooms, our shelters and soup kitchens, parishes and schools. We bring a human perspective in an often technical debate.

C. A third major asset we bring is a significant *capacity for advocacy*. We are not new to this debate. We have a potentially powerful constituency. We're present in every state and congressional district. We bring expertise and credibility rooted in our experience and values. Last year, we saw just an indication of our potential when we get our act together. Because of our size, presence, and principles, we can make a significant impact on health policy.

IV
An Agenda for Reform

I believe we must continue to offer a distinctive and constructive Catholic contribution to what will be one of the major social policy debates of our times. In this new environment, we continue to advocate the four priorities lifted up by the bishops' resolution.

1. *Universal Access/Priority for Poor.* Health care reform must put the needs of the poor and unserved first. Universal access must not be significantly postponed, since coverage delayed may well be coverage denied. Concrete steps toward universal access must be the centerpiece of health policy. Particular concerns for us are coverage for the uninsured and undocumented. Health care reform must be clearly measured by how it improves care for those now without coverage. It also should be judged by whether it improves or worsens care for undocumented and legal immigrants. Coverage of undocumented workers is important not only for moral reasons, but also for public health and cost containment reasons.

From the policy perspective, universal coverage is not only morally right, it is also needed to achieve some rational use of our health care resources. Many of the uninsured are not eligible for Medicaid and many work at jobs which do not offer health insurance and do not pay enough for the individual to purchase it. If you are uninsured, you sometimes can get medical care but only through an emergency room where the care is most expensive and least effective. Without universal coverage, cost shifting will continue and fewer people will be paying more for less health care coverage. Catholic health care institutions will also be jeopardized as money is taken from government programs to fund inadequate subsidies or to achieve deficit reduction.

The combination of a new political climate, less friendly to health care reform, the effects of a balanced budget amendment, and the certainty of Medicaid and Medicare cuts and entitlement caps, will likely have serious consequences for poor families and children. We must work to protect the weak. The sick and vulnerable cannot be abandoned. And in this new situation, we will work to protect and improve the coverage people now have and we will support incremental reform, if it represents clear progress toward our broader health priorities. For example, the nation should expand coverage for pregnant women and children in a way that would serve their health needs and make a down payment on universal coverage. As bishops, we are more clear about ends than means. We are not advocates of a specific plan, but of the need to restructure the health care system so that government, the private sector, and the voluntary community work together to assure decent health care for all.

2. *Respect for Life.* Health care reform must clearly protect life, not threaten it. Our Conference has insisted that it would be a moral tragedy, serious policy misjudgment, and major political mistake to burden health care, even in incremental reform measures, with abortion coverage. On this key issue we have public opinion with us and stronger support in the new Congress.

There are encouraging signs that both the American people and Congress recognize that there is something fundamentally wrong with coercing pro-life Americans to pay for the destruction of unborn children. We have made this case clearly and consistently and we must continue to do so. We still believe it politically unwise and morally wrong to burden health care with abortion mandates and to compel millions of people to fund what we believe is destruction of life, not healing and health care. This remains a fundamental criteria for health policy.

3. *Pursuing the Common Good and Preserving Pluralism.* We have learned all too clearly that reform can be undermined by special interest conflict. We believe future debates should be refocused on the common good and a healthy respect for genuine pluralism. A reformed system must encourage the creative and renewed involvement of both the public and private sectors, including voluntary, religious, and non-profit providers of care. It must also respect the religious and ethical values of both individuals and institutions involved in the health care system. A major priority

is protecting the non-profit role in health care delivery. We are deeply concerned that Catholic and other institutions with strong moral foundations are already facing increasing economic and regulatory pressures to compromise their moral principles. There must be strong protections so that Catholic institutions can serve the undocumented, protect unborn life, and follow religious teaching in their health ministry.

4. *Restraining Costs.* Health care policy must include effective mechanisms to restrain rising health care costs. By reducing health care inflation we could cut the federal deficit, improve economic competitiveness, and help stem the decline in living standards for many working families. Without cost containment, we cannot hope to make health care affordable and direct scarce national resources to other pressing problems which, in turn, worsen health problems (e.g., inadequate housing, poverty, joblessness, and poor education). Containing costs is a crucial task if we are to avoid the growing pressure for rationing that raises fundamental ethical and equity questions. The poor and vulnerable should not be denied needed care because the health system cannot eliminate waste, duplication, and bureaucratic costs.

In pursuing these priorities last year, now and in the future, I believe we unite the Catholic community. Our agenda is pro-life and pro-health care. Our criteria is focused on the unserved, uninsured, and unborn. We bring together our principles and our experience in a positive and consistent case for health care policy which enhances the life and dignity of all. The role of Catholic moral leadership in the health care arena should not be underestimated. The increasing complexity of bioethical issues (including issues at the beginning and ending of life, reproductive technologies, human experimentation) and the equally complex social justice issues (the right to health care, the breadth of universal coverage, etc.) require a consistent and coherent articulation of the Christian vision of the sacredness of life, human dignity, and the preferential option for the poor.

In response to these challenges, the Bishops' Conference has joined with the Catholic Health Association, the Leadership Conference of Women Religious, the Major Superiors of Men and Catholic Charities, USA, and others to form the National Coalition for Catho-

214

lic Health Care Ministry. Just last year, the National Conference of Catholic Bishops formed the Ad Hoc Committee for Health Care Issues and the Church to serve as episcopal liaison to the National Coalition. This bishops' committee, headed by Bishop Wuerl, will work with the coalition to examine the development of parish-based health care ministry and to provide guidance in addressing the issues of mergers, networking, and other partnerships between Catholic and non-Catholic health care services. These issues have been and will continue to be an important issue given the accelerating trend toward increased collaboration at every level of health care delivery.

In addition, as you undoubtedly know, at the November 1994 General Meeting of bishops, the revised *Ethical and Religious Directives* were unanimously approved. The new directives differ in their focus on service rather than facilities. In terms of mergers, the new directives call for involvement of diocesan bishops in any joint ventures, and require that diocesan bishops approve any such arrangements. They represent a major asset in reflecting Catholic identity and mission in health care.

In our ongoing advocacy, and these other efforts, our Conference will continue to work to help shape a health care system that will protect the unborn, reach out to the unserved and underserved, and contain costs and respect pluralism. It will be a long, tough, and complicated process. We need your help. It is not always easy to stand up for the unborn and undocumented, for uncovered children and uninsured families, but it is our duty.

V
Conclusion

As our Conference said eighteen months ago, health care reform "is a matter of fundamental justice. For so many, it is literally a matter of life and death, of lives cut short and dignity denied. We urge our national leaders to look beyond special interest claims and partisan differences to unite our nation in a new commitment to meeting the health care needs of our people, especially the poor and vulnerable. This is a major political task, a significant policy challenge, and a moral imperative."

While others may turn away from difficult issues when it becomes politically expedient to do so, we cannot. Our teaching on human life and health care and our commitment to the healing ministry of Jesus require the Church to continue to lift up this matter of great moral importance.

I've spoken a long time. Let me conclude with three brief summary points. *What happened last year?* The country didn't really have a dialogue about health care. Instead, we watched a debate dominated by partisan posturing and special interest pleading which left the country fearful and divided on health care reform. We haven't yet faced the crisis.

What does it mean? The problems of lack of access and rising costs remain with all their moral and human consequences. Reform will be likely be incremental and painful, but it is inevitable. The question remains what values and vision will guide this process.

What should we do? We must keep faith with our teaching on human life and health care. We should bring together our values, experience, and community in persistent and principled advocacy. We are called to stand with the poor and vulnerable, the unborn and uninsured. We must continue to make the case for genuine health reform that respects human life, enhances human dignity, and advances the common good.

Notes

1 *Pacem in Terris*, art. 11.
2 Encyclical Letter, *Centesimus Annus*, 1 May 1991, par. 10-11.
3 Ibid., par. 22, 34.

Chapter 15

THE PRINCIPLES OF COOPERATION AND THEIR APPLICATION TO THE PRESENT STATE OF HEALTH CARE EVOLUTION

The Reverend Russell E. Smith, S.T.D.

The virtually absolute silence of contemporary moral theologians regarding the application of the principles of cooperation to the present state of health care evolution and partnerships probably derives from their keen historical instincts. It was, after all, the nascent articulation of these principles by great casuists, such as Thomas

217

Sanchez and Tommaso Tamburini, that brought about the first intervention of the Magisterium in the field of morals. In 1679, Pope Innocent XI—through the agency of the Inquisition—condemned sixty-five theses of laxist moral doctrine. Number 51 is a laxist rendering of the sinfulness of a certain kind of cooperation.[1] It would take almost a century to articulate a coherent understanding of cooperation that was considered neither lax nor rigorist. This development would be fundamentally the work of St. Alphonsus Liguori.[2]

This presentation will be five-fold: a brief introduction of the horizon of moral life in relation to which the principles of cooperation make sense; a brief review of the different types of cooperation; theological and pastoral concerns regarding health care partnerships; the specific principles the Pope John Center is using in its consultation service to systems and dioceses; and finally an application to four large "arenas" of partnerships with special attention to three forms of alliances.

1. The Theological Horizon

The teaching of Christ and therefore the teaching of the Church has an ethical component.[3] Far from teaching the mere avoidance of evil action, Christ taught that one must be perfect as our heavenly Father is perfect (cf. Mt 5,48). Essentially, the moral aspect of the teaching of Christ requires serious asceticism involving prayer, fasting, and the cultivation of the virtues.

The practice of Christian faith has always forbidden the deliberate performance of evil acts. Evil acts, called sins, involve the violation of the law of God revealed in holy Scripture or in one's "heart" or conscience (cf. Rom 1, 20-32). The Christian religion strictly forbids the performance of an evil action even if good can come from it (Rom 3, 8).

This teaching, that the end does not justify the means, is not confined to the moral law of revealed doctrine. It is part of the patrimony of philosophical ethics. Socrates is the outstanding teacher of moral philosophy and this conviction is a cornerstone of his own ethics (cf. Plato's *Crito*). Socrates also taught that the performance of evil, the lack of morality, is itself the greatest ill one can suffer (cf. Plato's *Gorgias*). A line from Aristotle (the pupil of Plato) eulogizing Socrates concisely summarizes the role and goal of philosophical ethics: "This is the man whom evil men do not even have the right to praise, who taught us to be happy while being good."

Three concepts have been formulated and refined to deal with the ethical permissibility of actions which relate to either physical evil or the moral evil of other agents. These are known as (1) the principle of the double effect; (2) the choice of the "lesser evil"; and (3) the principles of cooperation. These concepts have been taught and reflected upon, and with the exception of (2), they have enjoyed unquestioned acceptance in philosophical ethics and Catholic moral theology. The precise formulations of these principles have varied from one school to another.

Underlying the tradition's formulations of these principles is unquestioned acceptance of an objective moral order and the conviction that some actions are "intrinsically evil," that is, are never justifiable regardless of the circumstances of the act. This is one of the major teachings of *Veritatis Splendor*. Proportionalism in general rejects both of these underlying presuppositions which necessitate the formation of the principles to begin with. At root, there is a fundamental disagreement between the Magisterium and proportionalists over the precise meaning of "the moral act." This question, while pivotal, is beyond the scope of this paper.

Proportionalism and its rejection or radical modification of the principles of double effect and cooperation is not acceptable as a basis of institutional protocol because the practical conclusions are generally in dissent from the teaching of the Church and are contrary to the clear teachings of Christ. Therefore, it is incumbent upon Catholic health care facilities and medical schools to evaluate procedures, protocols, and projects which concern physical and moral evil in light of the applicability of the principles of the double effect and cooperation.

2. The Principles of Cooperation

The precise question here is: What are the principles of cooperation and what bearing do they have on the present state of the evolution of health care delivery?

St. Alphonsus made the principles of cooperation acceptable by introducing the distinction between formal and material cooperation (the former never acceptable and the latter possibly acceptable) and by a consideration of scandal as a serious invitation to sin. It should be noted that since his time, many different moralists have made refinements and distinctions of their own, but the basic teaching derives from that of St. Alphonsus.[4]

Cooperation in the ethically significant sense is defined as the participation of one agent in activity of another agent to produce a particular effect or joint activity. This becomes ethically problematical when the action of the primary agent is morally wrong.

There are three basic examples of cooperation on the part of individuals: the hostage, the taxpayer, and the accomplice. The participation or cooperation of these individuals in the morally questionable acts of the principal agent is quite distinct one from another.

The hostage is forced to comply with the evil act of another person with threats. Fear of threatened harm on the part of the cooperator more or less compels the hostage to cooperate. This diminishes the culpability of the hostage and in some cases diminishes it completely. The new ERDs call this circumstance "duress" and duress renders the cooperation of the threatened party immediate material cooperation.

The accomplice may perform the same act as the hostage. But culpability is imputed fully in the case of the accomplice because cooperation in this instance is free and willed (directly intended).

The taxpayer is an example of one who cooperates with a principal agent (the government) in an important, in fact essential, mission (societal governance). Nevertheless, it is possible that the government sponsors activities which are immoral. The taxpayer contributes in some way to this immoral activity.

It is obvious at this point that the theological development of the principles of cooperation has considered the actions of *individuals* who cooperate with the evil actions of others. Contemporary theological considerations are not so insular. There are questions about "corporate actions" of cooperation, such as joint ventures between health care institutions in which the joint venture may be morally questionable because the philosophy and action of one of the partner institutions may be repugnant to the other cooperative institution. It should be remembered that not all, and in fact very few, acts of the non-Catholic partner are morally wrong, and the rest quite good. Their provision of health care is not intrinsically evil. That is why the analogy of the taxpayer to describe cooperation with them is so apt.

A complicating factor here is the fact that "cooperation" between institutions or systems is an arrangement made on the level of a legal corporation. The cooperative venture has a very precise and clearly defined identity and purpose, which may not be evident in the public forum. Media use language in a way that may actually misrepresent the nature of the partnership. The point here is this: the partnership is a legal and/or corporate structuring intended to perform only functions (1) which are mutually agreeable to all partners; (2) which do not include any procedures which any partner disagrees with on moral grounds; and (3) which explicitly separate the partnership from activities in which an individual partner may continue to engage.

Why is this sort of partnering necessary? There are several reasons. First, clinical medicine has reduced the need for the number of hospital beds that presently exist. Many procedures are handled on an out-patient basis, and more complicated procedures require a shorter hospital recovery period. Rehab Centers, long-term care facilities, and home care are alternatives for recuperation in acute care settings. Also, in the health care market, competition is a cost-driving factor, not a cost-containing force. What health care providers now compete for are not beds, but physicians (particularly primary care physicians who make referrals to other professionals and institutions) and patient markets (purchasers and consumers). The need to down-size acute care settings and create state of the art diagnostic and day treatment centers has led to the realization that health care must be cast in another form, which is often referred to as "rationalizing" care. The arena of rationalization includes health care alliances, joint ventures, physician organizations, and insurance products, which will be examined shortly.

221

The practical conclusion to this re-configuration is that a "stand alone" position is not always a viable option. In most cases it is foreseen that isolation would entail eventual closure. This market pressure is considered to be the "sufficient reason" which is one of the "ingredients" necessary to justify material cooperation.

The distinctions of cooperation may be recalled from one's seminary studies: the primary distinction is between formal and material cooperation. Formal cooperation is a willing participation on the part of the cooperative agent in the sinful act of the principal agent. The revised *Ethical and Religious Directives* make an interesting distinction between explicit and implicit formal cooperation (this distinction is rare in the manuals of moral theology):

> If the cooperator intends the object of the wrongdoer's activity, then the cooperation is formal and, therefore, morally wrong. Since intention is not simply an explicit act of the will, formal cooperation can also be implicit. Implicit formal cooperation is attributed when, even though the cooperator denies intending the wrongdoer's object, no other explanation can distinguish the cooperator's object from the wrongdoer's object. (ERDs, Appendix)

The motto of the implicit formal cooperator is "I am personally opposed, but…."

Material cooperation has several inherent distinctions, the most basic being that of immediate and mediate material cooperation. For Dominican Fathers McHugh and Chelan,[5] in the objective order, immediate material cooperation is equivalent to implicit formal cooperation because the object of the moral act of the cooperator is indistinguishable from that of the principal agent. They put it this way:

> Formal cooperation is implicit, when the cooperator does not directly intend to associate himself with the sin of the principal agent, but the end of the external act (*finis operis*), which for the sake of some advantage or interest the cooperator does intend, includes from its nature or from circumstances the guilt of the sin of the principal agent. Examples: Balbus detests idolatry, but in order to show courtesy he helps a pagan to burn incense before an idol, or he assists in the repairing of a pagan shrine, though his act is looked on as a sign of worship.[6]

While agreeing with this in principle, the new ERDs go on to say that

> Material cooperation is immediate when the object of the cooperator is the same as that of the wrongdoer. Immediate material cooperation is wrong, except in some instances of duress. The matter of duress distinguishes immediate material cooperation from implicit formal cooperation. But immediate material cooperation—without duress—is equivalent to implicit formal cooperation and, therefore, is morally wrong.

What the ERDs are trying to say here, I think, is that if an act of this sort of cooperation is freely done (as in the case of Balbus) it is implicit formal cooperation. If it is done under "duress" (such as driving a get-away car with a gun to one's head), it is immediate material cooperation. This precise distinction is not widely used in the tradition inasmuch as, morally speaking, the former is voluntary, the latter is non-voluntary (like the hostage). The manuals used *either* the language of implicit formal cooperation *or* immediate material cooperation to say the *same* thing, not two different things.[7] The ERDs do not elaborate on what constitutes duress for an institution as opposed to an individual. It seems to me that duress should be understood as episodic, not systemic. Otherwise, for example, protocols that would be sought to deal with alleged systemic duress to perform sterilizations would entail implicit formal cooperation.[8] My point is that the duress suffered by individuals is episodic and rare and that this part of the analogy should hold for institutions also.

Be that as it may, immediate material cooperation is contrasted with *mediate* cooperation. Here the moral object of the cooperator's act is not that of the wrongdoer's. This kind of cooperation can be justified for a sufficient reason (mentioned above) and if scandal can be avoided (which will be mentioned below). It is a form of cooperating with the circumstances surrounding the wrongdoer's act. Depending on how closely these circumstances impinge upon the act, there is a distinction between *proximate* and *remote* material cooperation. Further, *necessary* material cooperation is that without which the sinful act could not occur (e.g., opening a bank vault for a robber who had no explosives). *Contingent* cooperation (also called *free* cooperation) is that without which the evil act would still take place (e.g., opening the bank vault for a robber with explosives).[9]

The upshot is: formal cooperation is never permitted. Mediate material cooperation *may* be permitted if the act is not sinful itself, if there is a proportionately serious reason for doing so, and if scandal can be avoided.

A word about scandal: It is not the same as a Public Relations problem. Scandal is the leading of another to sin because one's actions either make evil seem good (or indifferent) or make evil seem like an attractive object. St. Thomas taught that scandal is "any word or deed not fully upright which is the occasion of sin to another." Father Ludovico Bender, O.P., of the Angelicum writes that

> While it is always sinful to give active scandal, in instances of passive scandal no sin is committed, if scandal proceeds from ill will, which sees an occasion of sin in conduct otherwise correct [i.e., Pharisaical scandal]; or if this scandal comes, due to the ignorance, lack of education, or moral formation of another, from an act, either not sinful in itself or necessary for the attainment of a good whose importance justifies our behavior. In such cases, there is no sin of scandal whatsoever.[10]

Therefore, while the formation of a partnership may pose public relations challenges, they are not necessarily constitutive of scandal.[11]

3. Theological/Pastoral Concerns vis-à-vis Health Care Partnerships

Needless to say, a determination that a proposed partnership is remote material cooperation is not the same as saying such a proposal is prudent. There may be local factors which complicate such an enterprise which the principles, baldly stated, would be blind to. This is the difficulty of prudential decisions in general. Ethical propriety does not mandate a particular course of action in this regard (as is characteristic of the positive precepts which bind "semper sed non pro semper").

In general, however, there are four basic theological and pastoral concerns that must be addressed. The extent and type of cooperation entailed in the partnership should be fleshed out. Cooperation with partners who perform some activities we deem morally inappropriate must derive from some "serious reason" or "moral necessity." As we saw, market pressures can be this serious reason. The potential for scandal–and the potential for notoriety–have to be looked at. As Dean Cafardi has shown us, the canonical questions of sponsorship and alienation of property require serious attention.

4. Five Basic Principles

There are five basic principles the Pope John Center is using as guidelines in moral evaluations of partnerships:

1. Cooperation must be mediate material, never formal or immediate material.

2. We can only do together what all partners agree to be appropriate. This means that while the alliance or collaborative effort need not be Catholic, it must nevertheless observe the ERDs as respecting the "corporate conscience" of the Catholic partner.

3. Morally illicit procedures cannot be provided on the Catholic campus.

4. Any morally illicit procedure(s) provided on campuses of non-Catholic alliance partners must be excluded from the new alliance corporation through separate incorporation and separate billing mechanisms.

5. All publicity should be straightforward regarding: (a) the need to form an alliance for survival of the apostolate; (b) the good achieved by "rationalizing" healthcare (the cost-driving reality of competition); (c) the exclusion of immoral procedures from the partnership (while these services will still be available on the campuses of some partner[s]); and (d) the necessity of this publicity appearing also in the promotional literature of the Catholic hospital.

5. Application to Models of Alliances

Alignments or affiliations take on four broad forms. (Others may develop.) The complexity of affiliations derives from the precise, concrete individuating circumstances of each alliance. However, *four basic forms are discernible.*

Form One: Contractual Relations Between Free Standing Institutions

This is the simplest form of cooperation. Precisely defined relationships are made by contract between free-standing institutions to do any of a number of things: e.g., provide pharmaceuticals or laundry service; concentrate neurology in one hospital or cardiology in another; etc. Generally, this is not morally significant.

This simple contractual relationship can also occur when separately sponsored hospitals join together to create a holding company which would rationalize care throughout several institutions. This is morally significant inasmuch as some elements of governance may pass from the realm of sponsorship to the new holding company. This may or may not also involve alienation of property. This stands at the vague borderline demarcating purely and precisely contractual relationship from greater inter-institutional cooperation characteristic of the Integrated Delivery Network.

Form Two: The Integrated Delivery Network (IDN)

This is a broad affiliation of providers and institutions across the entire spectrum of health care. This is a precisely cooperative venture with moral significance inasmuch as most IDNs involve non-Catholic partners who provide services prohibited by the ERDs. Catholic providers can participate in such affiliations if there is a serious reason or moral necessity, if the cooperation is mediate material, and if scandal can be avoided.

IDNs do not ordinarily involve alienation of property. While other partners in the IDN do not have to share the Catholic philosophy of health care ethics, partners should be selected who are not inimical to the Church's ethical standards. Networking can and does occur with institutions that provide a full range of reproductive services that would be unconscionable in a Catholic hospital.

Ethicists evaluate IDNs to be forums of material cooperation (of varying proximity) which can be justified only by a detailed examination of each case and its circumstances. Decisions involving the principles of cooperation require prudential judgments.

While bishops and many Catholic healthcare sponsors see the real wisdom of Catholic health care services joining among themselves first (e.g., Chicago), alliances of Catholic and non-Catholic health care facilities are occurring all over the country. It seems to be part of the natural evolution of the delivery of health care at this time. The exact shape that these alliances will take is impossible to predict. Some will provide a comprehensive range of health care services, others may merely redistribute services by abolishing costly duplication based on a former model of competition. However, the legislative *mandate* to create alliances or networks is no longer being emphasized. Therefore, some of the present impetus to create large IDNs *may* be reduced. However, it must be noted that alliances of some sort, i.e., affiliations which make health care less costly by reducing duplication of services and by responding to the lessened need for acute care bed space, will continue to take place in the market for the foreseeable future.

Form Three: The Purchase of Professional Services

Hospitals frequently purchase all or part of physicians' services. If one owns 100% of a physician's practice, the sponsor can mandate observance of the ERDs. Otherwise, the part owned by the Catholic sponsor can maintain this mandate only for that part of the practice it owns. Physicians are otherwise free to do what they will with the other X% of their practice. This has been done creatively in Peoria.

Form Four: The Creation of an Insurer

This is one of the most difficult forms of cooperation to determine. The creation of an HMO or other insurer/purchaser of health care would probably allow for services that could not take place in the Catholic facility. This is so either because the market "necessitates" this or because the government will mandate a basic benefits package which will require provision of all services. The question becomes two-fold: can a Catholic sponsor be a minority owner? and, can a Catholic sponsor be a majority owner?

The moral question is: can cooperation remain material in either or both cases? Ethicists are divided over this question. Of the *very* few who are writing/thinking/talking about this problem, there is emergent opinion that minority status is permissible since it remains (proximate, contingent, mediate) material cooperation if, as in the case of IDNs, separate incorporation of the prohibited procedures can isolate the Catholic partners from participation in the provision of prohibited services. The reasons for this will be mentioned in the resolution of the question of majority ownership, below.

Majority partnership would be at least immediate material cooperation which the tradition has not permitted, e.g., if sterilization services are offered in the benefits package. It is thought that the exclusion of sterilization from an insurance plan would make the plan unattractive and largely unmarketable. The question some ask is whether "immediate material" is an adequate evaluation of this cooperation. This is unresolved.

I would venture this opinion: In light of the five principles enunciated above, I think it is possible for a Catholic sponsor to be a majority owner of an HMO or an insurer if a separate, non-Catholic corporation were to be the underwriter or third party administrator for the prohibited procedures, made available to clients through the vehicle of a "rider" to their insurance policy. The Catholic sponsor would neither benefit from nor be liable for the weal or woe of sterilizations.

What are the moral realities here? The "moral object" of the Catholic provider is the provision of health care as a Gospel mission. It is providing for that mission in accord with its conscience. Some would say (and this will appear in print within the next few months) that even designing a way to "off-load" sterilizations is tantamount to making provision for the prohibited procedures: in a word, what this amounts to is immediate material cooperation.

"*Distinguo, salva reverentia.*" The moral object of creating an HMO is precisely *not* to provide prohibited procedures, *not necessarily to abolish them*. Prohibited procedures are part of the culture of America. In that sense, we live in a milieu of *toleration*, which is not *acceptance*. The rider to the insurance policy requires the client to go beyond *our* provision of health services. Since our intention is *not* to provide services we deem immoral, cooperation seems to be *material*. Because the client must choose to go beyond the basic health care plan, the material cooperation seems to be *mediate*–like providing for the transfer of a patient who wishes to leave our hospital "against medical advice." The mediate material cooperation seems to be *proximate* since the rider is designed by the Catholic sponsor. And finally, the proximate mediate material cooperation seems to be *contingent* since the prohibited procedures would continue even if the Catholic sponsor ceased to exist. A Catholic HMO designed this way will neither increase nor decrease the number of prohibited procedures. With careful crafting and publicity, it seems that this is able to be done.

Conclusion

In conclusion, the principles of cooperation are stated rather simply, explained with great difficulty, and applied with great angst. It is the angst of all pioneers into whatever frontier confronts one. Surely it was a condition known to Tamburini, Sanchez, and Alphonsus Liguori. And, as for them, so for us: our thoughts and theories are always subject to the judgment of the Magisterium. But these principles allow for great good to be done and great evil to be avoided.

Now that this claim has been staked on the frontier of health care partnerships, let the arrows fly!

Notes

1. See Denzinger and Schonmetzer [DS] 2101-2165, particularly 2151. The Decree in question concerns the opinion of Tommaso Tamburini, S.J., found in his *Explicatio decalogi* (Ludg. 1659) lib. V. cap. 1, no. 4. 19. The decree of the Holy Office of the Universal and Roman Inquisition, entitled "Errores doctrinae moralis laxioris" is of 2 March 1679, confirmed by His Holiness Pope Innocent XI as *Propositiones LXV damnatae*. Proposition no. 51 reads as follows: "Famulus, qui submissis humeris scienter adiuvat herum suum ascendere per fenestras ad stuprandam virginem, et multoties eidem subservit deferendo scalam, aperiendo ianuam, aut quid simile cooperando, non peccat mortaliter, si id faciat metu notabilis detrimenti, puta ne a domino male tractetur, ne torvis oculis aspiciatur, ne domo expellatur."

2. See Roger Roy, C.Ss.R., "La cooperation selon saint Alphonse de Liguori" *Studia Moralia*, 6: 377-435. This is a classic article which exhaustively reviews the development of this doctrine from Thomas Sanchez to St. Alphonsus.

3. This section of the paper is based in large part on my "The Principles of Cooperation in Catholic Thought" in *The Fetal Tissue Issue: Medical and Ethical Aspects*, ed. Albert S. Moraczewski, O.P., and Peter J. Cataldo (Pope John Center: Braintree, MA, 1994), 82, passim.

4. In some manuals of moral theology, St. Thomas Aquinas is cited as one of the first authors to reflect on the ethical aspects of cooperation. See *Summa Theologiae* II-II, 62, 7c which deals with cooperation in evil within the context of restitution. E.g., cf. Merkelbach *Summa Theologiae Moralis* (Third Edition, 1938), nos. 487-492.

5. J. A. McHugh, O.P. and C. J. Chelan, O.P., *Moral Theology* Volume I (London: Herder, 1958), nos. 1508-1546.

6. Ibid., no. 1511 (b).

7. Cf. M. Zalba, S.J., *Theologiae Moralis Summa*. Vol. I (Madrid: Biblioteca de Autores Cristianos, 1957), nos. 1606-1631, especially at 1609 (in which he says that an agent materially cooperates when the "cooperator does not intend the sin [of the principal agent], not even implicitly" ["per quam cooperator non intendit peccatum neque implicite"] without further explanation. And he continues [1611] that one does not formally cooperate when assistance is rendered with threats to one's life. This hostage situation is considered necessary mediate material cooperation.

8. On this precise point, see Charles Curran, "Cooperation in a Pluralistic Society" in *Ongoing Revision in Moral Theology* (Notre Dame: Fides/Claretian, 1975), 210-228. Also see his "Abortion: Its Legal and Moral Aspects" and "Sterilization: Exposition, Critique and Refutation of Past Teaching" both in *New Perspectives in Moral Theology* (Notre Dame: University of Notre Dame Press. 1974), 163-193 and 194-211, respectively. The point here is that the concept of "duress" is being used to make a practical necessity of sterilizations and abortions in Catholic hospitals. It is important to remember that this alleged practical necessity may be the fruit of theoretical rejection of the Church's teaching twenty years earlier.

9. This example is found in G. Atkinson and A. Moraczewski, O.P., *A Moral Evaluation of Contraception and Sterilization: A Dialogical Study* (St. Louis: The Pope John Center, 1979), 78-80.

10. Ludovico Bender, O.P., "Scandal" in *Dictionary of Moral Theology*, ed. Pietro Palazzini (Westiminster, MD: The Newman Press, 1962), 1096.

11. Directive 70 of the 1994 Revision of the *Ethical and Religious Directives for Catholic Health Care Services* reads as follows: "The possibility of scandal, e.g., *generating confusion about Catholic moral teaching*, is an important factor that should be considered when applying the principles governing cooperation. Cooperation, which in all other respects is morally appropriate, may be refused because of the scandal that would be caused in the circumstances" (Emphasis added). As stated, the italicized portion of this directive may be confusing to some readers because it does not precisely define scandal as "leading another into sin" or "making evil look good or attractive," but rather gives an example of one of the possible effects of active scandal.

Chapter 16

RESPONSE TO "THE PRINCIPLES OF COOPERATION AND THEIR APPLICATION TO THE PRESENT STATE OF HEALTH CARE EVOLUTION"

Sister Frances Marie Masching, O.S.F.

In a June 15, 1994 address, Pope John Paul II stated that the service of the sick "is a way of sanctification." He continued, "Down the centuries, it has been a manifestation of the love of Christ, who is precisely the source of holiness." When the Pope uses the expression "down the centuries," he reminds us of the permanent and enduring relationship of care that characterizes the profession of service to the sick.

We in Catholic health care maintain this faith-filled vision of enduring realities which is facing serious challenges at the present time. This is so because we are in a time of dramatic reconfiguration in health care in the United States. While it is certainly too early to tell whether there is true reform and improvement of health care access and delivery, there are many and frequent changes. In my years of service in Catholic health care, there has never been a time of such fundamental shifts in the structure of health care providers.

The rapidity of change is such that we often cannot wait for all the signs of a shift to be manifested—such would make our health care progress and facilities too late in adaptation. Health care systems are like large sea-going vessels; it takes a lot of time to make a turn. As a result, the OSF Healthcare System Board has advisors to assist us in making the many prudential judgments necessary in these troubled waters of change. It is imperative that our consultants and advisors understand our mission of service and our Catholic values as they make proposals regarding Board action. Advisors need to be educated well into the Mission.

The latest expression everyone in health care is using today is "vertically integrated networks." It is of recent coinage and basically refers to the continuum of treatment and care services, most of them *not* hospital based. Health care is shifting from the hospital to a continuum of care from conception to the end of life on earth. In many service areas today, forecasts of the future of health care tell providers that their future is bleak if they remain isolated as stand-alone hospitals. And there are many variations of joint venture or other networking arrangements proposed in health care.

Although the Catholic providers certainly face the same reconfiguration challenges of secular providers, we have our most important concerns as well. Specifically, although Catholic health care has to be part of this reconfiguration of health care to give the best guarantee of continuing the ministry to the sick, the injured, the aged, the dying, and the poor, our primary concern is with the continuing of a Catholic apostolate.

With respect to our situation, the Sisters of the Third Order of St. Francis, of Peoria, Illinois, of which I am a member, believe our stewardship of the Mission entrusted to us by the Church, in those instances in which a joint venture is considered, is to maintain the Catholic *Ethical and Religious Directives* in all the activities of the joint venture. Anything other than operation of the joint venture under these Directives would jeopardize the Catholic identity of that partnership.

Looking to the future, our apostolate is one that will bear witness to the truth and sacredness of human life at all its stages. This witness will develop as euthanasia trends increase in our nation and a new philosophy of pragmatism extends to human life and health care.

The apostolate of health care is also challenged by the growth of the phenomenon of purely for-profit health care provision. In our time, there is an increasing number of these for-profit providers, some of whom hope to purchase Catholic and other not-for-profit facilities, in an attempt to dominate certain service areas. All of the not-for-profit providers are called to witness to our belief that health care represents a fundamental human value, that it is based on patient-centered care, and is not a mere commodity. As for-profits take over, our concern as a Catholic provider is the alienation of Church property every time a for-profit buys out another Catholic facility.

Because the communities of religious women and men who sponsor Catholic health facilities have changed with fewer members, we Sisters have many lay associates in leadership and other responsible management positions. We must keep our Mission clearly in focus for them and show that Catholic health care is a mission of service of the love of Christ, and not a business or industry. Of course, this mission of service has a sizeable financial component, but these sound business practices are truly a stewardship for the Mission. We are mission-driven, supported by this stewardship.

Also, with respect to our lay associates, and recognizing the need for continuing formation in the values of the Mission, OSF Healthcare System has developed a Ministry Development Program for its management staff. In 1988-1989, we put 88 of our Leadership Executives through the Program. This number included Board Members, Chief Executive Officers, Physicians, Assistant Administrators, and Corporate Directors. They each had eleven days of intense education, with instructions by our Sisters, not consultants. We learned early that the people who are responsible for "hands-on" activities—supervisors, directors and managers of our health care facilities—needed to also be educated. Consequently, as of today, five years later, we have put approximately 800 through the Program. A large capital investment for the System, but it is a positive investment, and we are able to meet the challenge of health care today because of its effect. We also have ongoing Ministry Development Program sessions for all of our employees at each health care facility.

Material Cooperation Issues

Questions involving material cooperation with evil present the most difficult situations for our Sisters, because we cherish the teaching of the Church, and only when reliable advisors point out the very serious risk posed to the Mission without the involvement will we consider it. We present this situation to Bishop John Myers, Diocese of Peoria, and to his Episcopal Vicar for Health Care, Monsignor Steven Rohlfs. In addition, Father Russell Smith and the staff of the Pope John Center have provided great assistance to us at these times, and also Bishop Garland of Marquette and Bishop O'Neill of the Rockford Diocese, and now Bishop Doran.

Now, occasions of material cooperation are, *first* of all, as Father Smith points out, only considered if done so by duress or grave threat to the well-being of the Mission. *Second,* any cooperation will only be material. We believe that structuring any degree of material cooperation requires constant monitoring of its implementation. We keep our Corporate Ethicist extremely busy with the start-up questions on the practicalities of implementation, as well as how they play out. We do not want to be part of the "slippery slope" syndrome.

The *third* consideration is that of scandal, which requires perpetual concern. The arrangements may be set up, but the danger of scandal to God's people can undo the most careful structure. This is another area in which our Ministry Development Program has been so helpful. As our managers go through this continuing formation program, they grow in awareness of the concerns the Church has in these matters, and, after five years of an intense program, we are at the point now where they recognize developing issues and problems so that we can deal with them in a timely manner. In these material cooperation issues, it is essential that managers and physicians throughout the facility or System be able to describe the Catholic provider's limited role and be able to explain the relationships in these arrangements.

OSF Healthcare System has very practical examples with our experience both in the development of a network of 102 primary care physicians and now a new HMO insurance product serving Central Illinois. As of January 1, 1995, we are the only Catholic HMO in the United States that is based on the *Ethical and Religious Directives* of the Catholic Church.

In the final analysis, we recognize that the people you have working with you will determine your success in dealing with these matters. If there is a short-changing or lack of true concern for the Church's moral teaching, that Catholic facility will have a hard time structuring and implementing any relationship involving material cooperation. Because our people are our greatest assets, I believe where you have associates of good will, who understand our concern, first of all, for the well-being of our Mission, we are much better equipped to face the challenges ahead.

These material cooperation issues are critical to Catholic identity. I can easily imagine cases in which a Catholic System can plan an arrangement that is remote material cooperation on paper, but, in practice, slips into the appearance of acceptance or promotion of immoral services. Such a situation would result in scandal and great harm to the Catholic people. Structuring these arrangements requires great care, both in the early stages and with the necessary follow-through and eternal vigilance regarding scandal. We could have never begun to implement a Catholic HMO for our System if we had not developed our Ministry Development Program and educated our lay associates. We believe they have been called to assist us in our apostolic endeavors.

It is also appropriate to foster collaboration among Catholic providers. This is assisted by a common mission from the Church, and common values relative to health care, concern for the poor, and the sacredness of human life. Any significant degree of collaboration, however, requires the two systems to also share a common sense of how they have to adapt to meet future health care reconfiguration. Common values may start the conversation, but a common sense of the future is also required. Ultimately, collaboration is a very practical activity.

Conclusion

This is a time of severe and continuing challenge to the Catholic health care mission, on so many levels. We who have been given this sacred mission of caring for the sick, the poor, and the dying, look to our pastors for a renewed dialogue on current developments. We welcome concern, interest and guidance on the place of Catholic health care in reevangelization, so that Catholic health care may not simply survive, but have a genuine renewal of our apostolate of service to the Church and a positive effect on all persons in need.

Chapter 17

RESPONSE TO "THE PRINCIPLES OF COOPERATION AND THEIR APPLICATION TO THE PRESENT STATE OF HEALTH CARE EVOLUTION"

Patricia A. Cahill, J. D.

As I read Father Smith's paper, I was impressed by the precision with which he describes the Principles of Cooperation and I was reminded of my own four-year preparation in theology and philosophy at Emmanuel College in Boston. I was, however, also somewhat disheartened by Father's description because it is my opinion that only a small percentage of the participants in our Catholic health and human service organizations truly grasp the principles which Father elucidated. And it is that lack of understanding, in my opinion, which is complicating so enormously the move by Catholic providers of health care to partner with non-Catholics.

The majority of joint ventures, networks, mergers and affiliations which have occurred and which are on the drawing board are, from my observation, driven from a business or economic perspective. The leaders responsible for consummating these arrangements understand the business world well. They also understand and support fully the fact that no proscribed services may be offered by their own Catholic institution. However, when the transaction under consideration is between the Catholic provider and a non-Catholic provider and its consummation promises improved fiscal well-being for the Catholic partner, attention sometimes shifts from strict adherence to the *Ethical and Religious Directives* to a tone of compromise which recognizes the ethical perspective of the non-Catholic provider and softens the principle to achieve the desired outcome. These are not people who intend to do wrong but they are people who have not necessarily had the theological and philosophical preparation to address appropriately the material cooperation questions before them. They hear the term "material cooperation" but do not understand its philosophical underpinnings and rationale and thus, in my opinion, are ill equipped to apply the principle to the matter at hand.

As Father Smith says, prudential judgment must be applied to each set of circumstances where a cooperative or collaborative effort is being made. I agree completely. My concern however, is simply that those exercising the prudential judgment often lack a sufficient basis from which to exercise their prudence and that those who possess the appropriate background are infrequently present at the negotiating table. However, let me add that if the bishop, the moral theologian, or ethicist is to be anywhere included in discussions, it is in the forum that relates to ethical and religious issues. It is generally conceded that there is a role to be played by the Church when such matters are discussed. Yet, in more generic business discussions that relate to joint venture, merger, affiliation, or network, the Ordinary or his representative is rarely present. A not uncommon opinion is that the Ordinary has no real role in such discussions when specifics of ethical and religious issues are not involved. The bishop is often relegated to the sole role of moral leader with the "deal makers" neither recognizing nor understanding the bishop's overriding concern and responsibility for the entire health care apostolate in the diocese. In my opinion, we desperately need education—a required education in moral theology and canon law—of our health care leadership to an awareness of what is at stake here, why it is important that it be protected, and the role of the Ordinary in assuring that protection.

Now that I've elaborated on my basic concern in this entire process, let me assure you that I am fully supportive of creatively investigating opportunities to partner with non-Catholic organizations. Let there be no mistake, my preference is that we partner with Catholic providers first because of the positive synergy that can be generated between partners who share a belief system. However, within today's health care environment, that is not always possible and the general benefit to a community of joint activity between its health care providers has to be seen as a "good" to be pursued. It is even more important that Catholic providers not "throw in the towel" and exit health care in this country. It's too large and important in the life of each person for the Church not to be appropriately represented within it. It offers an almost unparalleled opportunity to witness Christ's healing ministry, particularly to the poor, and on the firing line, to attest to the value of each human person. Certainly it is not an opportunity to be lightly sacrificed.

So, how do we remain in the arena, negotiate with possible partners, and develop accommodations which are not violative of our principles and which keep us within the appropriate boundaries of material cooperation? I'd like to offer descriptions of two projects which are evolving in the Archdiocese of New York.

The first is a Prepaid Health Services Plan, a joint venture between a Catholic hospital and a non-denominational clinic corporation. The purpose of this joint venture is to offer a managed care product to Medicaid recipients. For both providers, the Medicaid population represents a substantial part of their business. If each is to remain a viable provider of health care services in its community, each needs to continue to serve and to enlarge its Medicaid population base, and each needs a partner to supplement its present geographic and programmatic activity. Additionally, service to the Medicaid population addresses the Church's commitment to a preferential option for the poor.

Representatives from the Department of Health and Hospitals of the Archdiocese and a moral theologian were present for several of the negotiating sessions between the two parties as they developed this new effort. There was an attitude of cooperation present. Both parties wished to consummate the arrangement. It is important to note here that the fact that there is a large number of health care providers in the New York area may create a more comfortable compromise situation for a non-Catholic provider on issues which involve the principle of material cooperation. There appear to be many other ways in which clients or patients can access services which are proscribed within a joint venture in which the non-Catholic is combining with a Catholic provider.

In this case, the newly established joint venture will adhere to the *Ethical and Religious Directives for Catholic Health Services.* All enrollees will be advised that proscribed services are not available through the joint venture. The legal entitlement of enrollees to "assured access" to such services will be met by distribution of a comprehensive list of health care providers, and neither the Catholic hospital nor its non-Catholic clinic partner is on the list of providers given to patients seeking proscribed services. The non-Catholic provider did not, however, limit its services outside of the joint venture to those services which conform to the *Ethical and Religious Directives.*

A second illustration of this model in the Archdiocese of New York is the collaboration between a Catholic hospital and a non-Catholic hospital to create a new hospital entity, essentially "a hospital without walls." In effect, the two hospitals agree to plan jointly and, with the new entity, develop and implement "centers of excellence," to be located at one or the other of the two hospital campuses. The two hospitals jointly and equally control the new entity. Like the Medicaid managed care organization described above, the new entity abides by the *Ethical and Religious Directives* and the non-Catholic partner does not limit its services outside of the joint venture to those services which conform to the Directives. This situation describes the classic two hospital town where the town's benefit derives from the cooperation of its two health care facilities since both cannot be sustained and neither wishes to leave the market.

In both of these situations, scandal is a possibility and good, clear information is important for sharing with multiple communities: patients, employees, and the public. We need to communicate the good we are attempting to achieve:

- An improved continuum of care to a Medicaid population by a Catholic provider;

- A less costly, better coordination of service in a two hospital town

We need to communicate simply the legal and corporate structure we have employed to achieve the "good" objective. This isn't an easy assignment. Often people don't understand the subtle nuances of these arrangements. But these are hard times in health care generally, and for our purposes, in Catholic health care particularly.

As integrated delivery networks evolve, we are likely to find ourselves increasingly in partnership with non-Catholic providers in a wide variety of organizational arrangements. Without a dominant position in such a network, there is always the threat we will lose control of our own destiny. However, if we are to emerge in the next century as a major player in the health care field, organizational and programmatic creativity which is also faithful to our moral and ethical tradition is demanded of us today. I think that Catholic healthcare providers are so important to the debates likely to rage around medical/moral issues in health care that we must keep trying to find acceptable answers and workable models, while exercising our prudential judgment.